Here's How Children Learn Speech and Language

A Text on Different Learning Strategies

Here's How Series

Thomas Murry, PhD
Series Editor

Here's How Children Learn Speech and Language: A Text on Different Learning Strategies by Margo Kinzer Courter

Here's How to Treat Childhood Apraxia of Speech by Margaret A. Fish

Here's How to Do Therapy: Hands-On Core Skills in Speech-Language Pathology by Debra M. Dwight

Here's How Children Learn Speech and Language

A Text on Different Learning Strategies

Margo Kinzer Courter, MBA, MA, CCC-SLP

Courter Communications, LLC
Indianapolis, Indiana

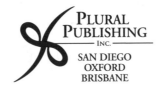

PLURAL
PUBLISHING
INC.

SAN DIEGO
OXFORD
BRISBANE

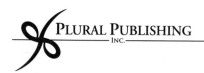

5521 Ruffin Road
San Diego, CA 92123

e-mail: info@pluralpublishing.com
Web site: http://www.pluralpublishing.com

49 Bath Street
Abingdon, Oxfordshire OX14 1EA
United Kingdom

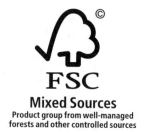

FSC
Mixed Sources
Product group from well-managed
forests and other controlled sources

Cert no. SW-COC-002283
www.fsc.org
© 1996 Forest Stewardship Council

Copyright © by Plural Publishing, Inc. 2011
Typeset in 11/15 Stone Informal by Flanagan's Publishing Services, Inc.
Printed in the United States of America by McNaughton and Gunn

Library of Congress Cataloging-in-Publication Data

Courter, Margo Kinzer.
  Here's how children learn speech and language : a text on different learning strategies / Margo Kinzer Courter.
      p. cm. — (Here's how series)
  Includes bibliographical references and index.
  ISBN-13: 978-1-59756-366-6 (alk. paper)
  ISBN-10: 1-59756-366-8 (alk. paper)
  1. Children with disabilities—Education. 2. Speech disorders in children. 3. Language disorders in children. 4. Response to intervention (Learning disabled children) I. Title.
  LC4015.C653 2011
  371.91'42—dc23
                           2011016911

Contents

CHAPTER 3   GETTING STARTED: PRELITERACY SKILLS   41

CHAPTER 4   READING IS ROCKET SCIENCE   69

CHAPTER 5   ACROSS THE CURRICULUM   89

CHAPTER 6   EXPRESSING ONESELF THROUGH WRITING   119

CHAPTER 7   PUBLISHERS PROVIDE WHAT?   135

CHAPTER 8   CLASSROOM STRATEGIES   141

CHAPTER 9   STRATEGIES FOR HOME   159

CHAPTER 10   THE GREATEST RESOURCES   171

Foreword

The "Here's How Series" is a collection of texts written as a 'hands on" approach to understanding and treating a specific disorder. This series emanated out of an observation that speech-language pathologists who work in varied environments, hospitals, clinics, school systems and private practice, were buyers of the book, *Here's How to Do Therapy* by Debra Dwight. Debra's unique "here's how" approach was intended primarily for young clinicians. However, records show that not only young clinicians but experienced clinicians, teachers, and students were also buying the book. Soon after the purchase of that book, however, clinicians were asking for a similar book but with more detail about specific topics—child language, autism, fluency, and literacy to name a few. This series offers exactly that—an in-depth approach to specific topics.

Each author in the "Here's How Series" is a clinician first and foremost in his or her area of speech-language pathology. Each brings years of experience with success to support that experience. You won't find extensive reference lists but you will find the author's well-documented and success driven practices to the topics discussed. You, the clinician, will find practical information to raise your clinical practice to the highest level. And you'll enjoy sharing the authors' experiences through the pages brought to life with case studies, case vignettes, and clinical tips based on the authors' experiences. We hope you enjoy Plural Publishing's "Here's How Series."

In Margo Courter's book, *Here's How Children Learn Speech and Language: A Text on Different Learning Strategies,* the author focuses on the critical steps in diagnosis before leading the clinician to the treatment details. Her chapter on "Just the Facts" provides exactly that, the essentials needed to navigate the diagnostic process. What to look for, how to assess it, and how to prioritize the treatment provide the groundwork without the need for extensive documentation, but with well-established treatment methods. The clinician is then given step-wise treatment protocols for written, spoken, and reading language. In the final section, Courter offers resources for the teacher and the student, along with classroom strategies to achieve the desired goals in language learning.

Thomas Murry, PhD
Series Editor

Preface

The purpose of this resource is to provide speech-language pathologist and educator information regarding language-based learning disabilities and strategies for academic success. Research tells us that 80% of students with learning disabilities also have a language disorder. Response to Intervention (RTI) calls for us to provide evidence-based differentiated instruction to struggling learners. I see many students who are not identified for special education services but are still struggling learners; therefore, they would not be included in these statistics.

The text provides background information regarding learning disabilities and the governing laws that ensure an appropriate education for all students and a call for evidence-based practices and differentiated learning. This text discusses how students with a language based learning disability are identified. Specific tests that can be used to determine the extent of the disability are discussed. The information provided in the diagnostic section mostly relates to the tests that a speech-language pathologist would use as part of an interdisciplinary team or would use independently outside of a school environment. The text then moves into what to do once a thorough evaluation is completed. It includes red flags that may be indicative of a language-based learning disability even when working with the youngest of preschool-age children. It also includes specific strategies that can be used from preliteracy skills through early reading. Because language exists across all areas of one's life and across all subject matters, strategies are provided regardless of the subject matter that the language-based learning disability is affecting. Classroom strategies and home strategies are presented as well. Lastly, Chapters 7 and 10 address what is now available through textbook publishers as well as other resources that provide great information that can be used in conjunction with what the textbook publishers offer.

The work environment for a child is school, and he or she must be successful in this work environment. Once the underlying diagnoses are obtained, the speech-language pathologist can identify goals as part of an overall intervention team.

The strategies presented in this tool will provide the speech-language pathologist and educator with ways to meet the student's speech/language goals while using strategies through what the child is learning in school. The strategies can be used across all curriculum areas for increased academic success.

I have used the strategies that are provided in this resource with many students with great success. It is exciting to watch students get excited about learning. An example I give in one of the chapters is about a soon-to-be eight grader I saw. During a school assignment where the students had to discuss the one thing that they wanted others to know about them that they may not already know, the student responded, "I read my first book this summer."

These are the powerful statements from our students that continue to motivate us to be part of the miracle of learning. I hope this book provides a resource to you, my colleagues, as you continue to provide invaluable services to those who so deserve it.

Margo Kinzer Courter, MBA, MA, CCC-SLP

*This work is dedicated to the following persons who have
shaped my life both professionally and personally:*

My husband, Bill, and sons, Brandon and Evan, as well as my parents,
Charlie and Lois Kinzer—Their support and encouragement through all of my
adventures provided the foundation to pursue my professional dreams.

My graduate school supervisor, mentor, colleague, editor and, above all, friend,
Kathryn "Katie" Smith, PhD, Speech-Language Pathologist—Her wisdom and support
continues to push me to be all that I can be as a speech-language pathologist.

All of the students and families I have been fortunate to serve—They provide
the motivation and the ah-ha moments that keep me pushing forward.

*Thanks to all,
Margo Kinzer Courter*

1

Just the Facts

Introduction

Imagine being a struggling student or a student with a diagnosed learning disability sitting in a classroom and hearing the teacher rave about others' work. Imagine seeing your sibling's excellent report card posted on the refrigerator. Imagine your siblings being honor roll students. Imagine hearing teachers and parents commenting, "Look at Lisa, she is always prepared and works so hard." "Why can't you be more like her?" "You just need to try harder." Imagine the constant red marks on papers for errors and incorrect responses. This may be a daily occurrence for the students with whom we are privileged to spend our day.

This chapter focuses on laying the groundwork for the information that is presented throughout this textbook. This includes some basic definitions that are further defined in other chapters. It also reviews the laws that govern the rights of those with disabilities, specifically those that affect students with learning disabilities, including language-based learning disabilities, which is the focus of this text.

Here Are Important Definitions

- *Accommodations*: Accommodations are tools and procedures that provide equal access to instruction and assessment for students with disabilities. This may include allowing answers to be given orally instead of in writing.

- *Americans with Disabilities Amendments Act of 2008 (ADAA)*: This law amends the Americans with Disabilities Act (ADA) and has a direct impact on Section 504 of the Rehabilitation Act.

- *Free appropriate public education (FAPE)*: FAPE is a significant cornerstone to the Rehabilitation Act and, specifically, Section 504 of this act. A child with a disability in the United States cannot be excluded from the participation in, be denied the benefits of, or be subjected to discrimination under any program or activity receiving federal financial assistance solely due to the disability.

- *Individuals with Disabilities Education Act of 2008 (IDEA 2008)*: IDEA 2008 is the latest reauthorization of IDEA and places further emphasis on a quick response when difficulties are noted with a student.

- *Language-based learning disability*: A language-based learning disability is described by the American Speech-Language-Hearing Association (ASHA) as problems with age-appropriate reading, spelling, and/or writing. This disorder is not about a person's intelligence (ASHA, n.d.).

- *Local education agency (LEA)*: LEA is the public board of education or other public authority within a state that maintains administrative control of public elementary or secondary schools in a city, county, township, and/or school district.

- *Learning disability*: A definition offered by LD OnLine (http://www.ldonline), a leading Web site on learning disabilities and attention deficit disorder, states that a learning disability is a neurological disorder. "In simple terms, a learning disability results from a difference in the way a person's brain is wired." Children with learning disabilities may have difficulty reading, writing, spelling, reasoning, recalling, and/or organizing information" (LD OnLine, n.d.).

The National Center for Learning Disabilities (NCLD) defines a student with a learning disability as one with at least average intellectual capacity. This student demonstrates a significant yet unexplained discrepancy between achievement and expected potential. A diagnosed learning disability excludes intellectual disabilities, emotional disturbance, cultural differences, or lack of opportunity to learn. Lastly, the center defines a learning disability as a central nervous system dysfunction as the basis of the presenting problem(s). The NCLD further explains that more than 2.5 million students are diagnosed with a learning disability and receive special education services in our schools (LD OnLine, 2011).

- *Mitigating measures*: Under the ADA, mitigating measures are defined as medications and assistive devices that an individual uses to eliminate or reduce the effects of impairment. Under ADAA 2008, mitigating measures can only be considered on a limited basis.

- *Modification*: A modification is a change in what is being taught to or expected from the student. This may include reducing the amount of homework or changing the format of a test.

- *No Child Left Behind Act of 2001 (NCLB)*: This law places greater accountability to identify and appropriately educate all students.

- *Response to Intervention (RTI)*: RTI is a tiered approach used to identify and provide intervention to students who may be struggling in certain academic areas.

- *Specially designed instruction*: Specially designed instruction is defined in IDEA as adapting the content, methodology, or delivery of instruction to address the needs of the student that result from the student's disability (Cohen, 2007).

- *Specific learning impairment (SLI)*: SLI is defined as a disorder in perceiving, understanding, and/or using concepts through spoken or written language or nonverbal means.

Here Are Some Facts

The following section offers some facts regarding learning disabilities.

Fact #1: Percent of Students With Learning and Language Disabilities

Research tells us that as many as 80% of students identified with a learning disability also have a language disability (Reed, 2005).

Fact #2: (Central) Auditory Processing Disorder (APD), Language Impairment, and Reading Disorder

Language impairment and reading disorders commonly co-occur with APD (Sharma, Purdy, & Kelly, 2009).

Fact #3: Childhood Apraxia of Speech, Language, and Learning Disorders

Children with Childhood Apraxia of Speech (CAS) may present with a comorbid language impairment, which places them at a higher risk for learning difficulties such as reading disorders (Lewis, 2007).

Fact #4: Word-Finding, Language Impairment, and Learning Disabilities

German (1998) and Dockrell, Messer, George, and Easton (1998) have stated that the prevalence of word-finding difficulties is high among learners with specific language impairment and learning disabilities.

Fact #5: Percent of Students With Learning Disabilities

According to the National Institutes of Health, 8% to 10% of children in the United States under the age of 18 have some type of learning disability (National Institutes of Health, 2010).

Fact #6: Language-Based Learning Disability Is a Better Descriptor Than Dyslexia

ASHA states that the term *dyslexia* has been used to refer to the specific learning problem of reading. However, the term *language-based learning disability*, or just *learning disabilities,* is a better description because of the relationship between spoken and written language. Many children with reading problems have spoken language problems as well (ASHA, n.d.).

Here Are Some Signs for Students Who May Be at Risk of a Learning Disability

The NCLD offers a checklist to identify students who are at risk for learning disabilities. It is in a brochure format. This checklist can be printed and used by parents and educators to assess risk factors for their students (NCLD, 2009).

ASHA also offers the following signs of a possible learning disability. The list includes signs for those with a possible language-based learning disability (ASHA, n.d.). The student may have difficulty:

- expressing ideas on paper
- understanding and retaining the details of a story's plot or a classroom lecture
- reading and comprehending material
- learning words to songs and rhymes
- listening and taking notes
- following oral and written instructions
- memorizing facts
- recalling numbers in a sequence
- retrieving known information
- organizing materials and ideas

Using a checklist of some type could be the first step in identifying students who may be struggling. It also may lead to appropriate intervention strategies and/or appropriate referrals for an interdisciplinary evaluation and appropriate treatment for the student.

In conclusion, I know that as I look at this list many language diagnoses come to mind. So if we refer back to the statistic that 80% of students with learning disabilities also have a language disorder, and we look at the list of signs, it is easy to start putting these two areas together for the term that is referred to throughout this text as *language-based learning disability*.

Here Are the Laws That Guarantee an Equal Education for All

Several federal laws guarantee equal education for all students. These are the Individuals with Disabilities Education Act (IDEA 2004), the No Child Left Behind Act of 2001 (NCLB), and Section 504 of the Rehabilitation Act. The newest law is an amendment to the ADA known as the Americans with Disabilities Amendments Act of 2008 (ADAA), which has a direct impact on the Rehabilitation Act and Section 504.

Introduction to Individuals With Disabilities Education Act (IDEA 2004)

IDEA has undergone several changes since its inception in 1975 as the Education for All Handicapped Children Act (EHA), or Public Law 94-142. This law originated as a way to ensure that students with disabilities received an appropriate public education. This law was reauthorized in 2008.

Twenty-one years ago, President Ford signed into legislation a law that was intended to improve opportunities in education for children and adults with disabilities through the provision of FAPE. This law was called EHA, or Public Law 94-142. It provided that children and adults ages 3 through 21 with a diagnosed disability be educated in the least restrictive environment to the maximum extent appropriate. Only students who demonstrated severe disabilities could be educated in special classes, special classrooms, or separate schools. The law has been updated approximately every 5 years. The latest revision is known as the Reauthorization of IDEA 2004, which was put into effect on December 31, 2008. A previous version of IDEA determined that disability was based on the discrepancy between intelligence quotient and achievement scores. Reauthorization of IDEA 2008 calls for closer monitoring of the curriculum; methods of teaching; and intervention strategies, rather than waiting for a referral for formal evaluation; and to determine if a student should be considered for special education (Sousa, 2007).

Here's Information Regarding Reauthorization of IDEA 2008

The reauthorization of IDEA 2004 (IDEA 2008) is designed to encourage school districts to provide additional support for struggling students within general education. The law calls for schools to intercede as soon as they observe a student struggle. Schools can no longer wait until a child is identified, permission is given for an evaluation, and a case conference is held to begin services for a student who is struggling. This support should be provided as early as possible—when students show the earliest signs of difficulty. This current approach is based on an improved, research process known as RTI.

Key Components of RTI

The following offers the key components to an RTI program. These are the elements that make up the tiered process for prompt intervention as soon as a student is recognized to be struggling (Sousa, 2007).

- Monitor a student's progress in the general curriculum using appropriate screenings or tests.

- Choose and implement scientifically proven interventions to address a student's learning problems.

- Follow formal guidelines to decide which students are not making sufficient progress or responding to the intervention.

- Monitor how the student responds to the intervention by using assessments at least once a week or once every 2 weeks.

- Make sure that the interventions are provided accurately and consistently.

- Determine the level of support that a student needs in order to be successful.

- Give parents notice of a referral and a request to conduct a formal evaluation if a disability is suspected.

Here Are the Benefits of RTI

There are many benefits to RTI. The use of an RTI process as part of a school's procedures for determining whether a student has a learning disability and needs special education services potentially can provide the following:

- Reduce the time a student waits before receiving additional instruction because the student will not have to wait for the evaluation process in order to receive services.

- Reduce the overall number of students referred for special education services and increase the number of students who succeed within general education.

- Ensure that students receive appropriate instruction, particularly in reading, prior to placement in special education.

Here's a Three-Tier RTI Model

RTI provides a framework for working with students as soon as difficulties arise. This may be difficulty with the day-to-day curriculum or it may be scores that are below the accepted cutoff on a universal screening used to measure mastery of skills at each grade level within specific time frames of each grade.

Tier 1: High-Quality Instruction, Screening, and Group Interventions

Students who are at risk may be identified using universal screenings and/or results on state- or district-wide tests. Identified students receive supplemental instruction or interventions generally delivered in small groups during the student's regular school day in the regular classroom. The length of time for this step can vary, but it generally should not exceed 8 weeks. During that time student progress is closely monitored. At the end of a specified period, students showing significant progress are generally returned to the regular classroom program. Students not showing adequate progress are moved to Tier 2.

Tier 2: Targeted Interventions Within General Education

Students not making adequate progress in the regular classroom in Tier 1 are provided with more intensive services and interventions. These services are provided in addition to instruction in the general curriculum. These interventions are provided in small group settings. In the early grades, kindergarten through third grade, interventions usually are provided in the areas of reading and behavior as well as possibly math. Parents are informed and included in the planning and monitoring at this tier. Students who continue to show too little progress at this level of intervention are then considered for more intensive interventions as part of Tier 3.

Tier 3: Intensive Interventions

At Tier 3, students receive individualized, intensive interventions that target the students' skill deficits. Students who do not respond to these targeted interventions are then considered for eligibility for evaluation and determination of a disability as required by the reauthorization of IDEA 2008. The data collected during Tiers 1, 2, and 3 are included, along with data from a comprehensive assessment. These are then used to make the eligibility decision for special education services. Parents are notified of their due process, and consent is gained for a comprehensive evaluation.

At any point in an RTI process, IDEA allows parents to request a formal evaluation to determine eligibility for special education. An RTI process cannot be used to deny or delay a formal evaluation for special education. For more information on IDEA provisions see NCLD's Parent Guide to IDEA at its Web site, LD.org, and read "Laws Protecting Students" (NCLD, n.d.).

Parentally Placed Private School Children With a Disability

IDEA is designed to improve educational results for all students with disabilities. This includes making provisions for students with disabilities enrolled by their parents in nonpublic (private) schools. The LEA's obligations to parentally placed private school students with disabilities are different.

Private School Plans for Parentally Placed Private School Children With a Disability

A private school plan must be developed and implemented for each private school student with a diagnosed disability. The LEA in which the private school is located is responsible for providing any services. The LEA must initiate and conduct meetings to develop, review, and revise a services plan for a child designated to receive services. The services plan must describe the specific special education and related services that the

LEA will make available to students of parentally placed private school children with disabilities. These services may include specific professionals who may provide services to the private school (e.g., speech-language pathologist) or other professionals who will provide consultation to the private school regarding the identified students (U.S. Department of Education, 2008).

Here's Information Regarding the NCLB Act of 2001

According to the Department of Education Web site, the NCLB Act of 2001, which reauthorizes the Elementary and Secondary Education Act of 1994 (ESEA), increased accountability for states, school districts, and schools. It offers greater choice for parents and students, particularly those attending low-performing schools, and more flexibility for states and LEAs in the use of federal education dollars. It also places a stronger emphasis on reading, especially for our youngest children (U.S. Department of Education, 2008).

Accountability Under NCLB

The NCLB Act also strengthens accountability by requiring states to implement statewide accountability systems covering all public schools and students. These systems must be based on state standards in reading and mathematics, annual testing for all students in Grades 3 through 8, and annual statewide progress objectives ensuring that all groups of students reach proficiency within 12 years. School districts and schools that fail to make adequate yearly progress (AYP) toward statewide proficiency goals will, over time, be subject to improvement, corrective action, and restructuring measures aimed at getting them back on course to meet state standards. Schools that meet or exceed AYP objectives or close achievement gaps will be eligible for state academic achievement awards (U.S. Department of Education, 2008).

Choices for Parents Under NCLB

The NCLB Act significantly increases the choices available to the parents of students attending Title I (certain percent of low-income students) schools that fail to meet state standards. LEAs must give students who are attending schools identified for improvement, corrective action, or restructuring the opportunity to attend a better public school, which may include a public charter school, within the school district. The district must provide transportation to the new school and must use at least 5% of its Title I funds for this purpose, if needed.

For students attending schools that do not make AYP, LEAs must permit low-income students to use Title I funds to obtain supplemental educational services from the public- or private-sector provider selected by the students and their parents (U.S. Department of Education, 2008).

Introduction to Section 504 of the Rehabilitation Act (1998)

According to the Department of Education, on September 23, 1973, Congress passed the Rehabilitation Act in response to federal lawsuits safeguarding the educational rights of children with disabilities. This act was the first federal civil rights law protecting the rights of those with disabilities. Among its many provisions, Section 504 declares that "No otherwise qualified individual with a disability in the United States shall, solely by reason of her or his disability, be excluded from the participation in, be denied the benefits of, or be subjected to discrimination under any program or activity receiving federal financial assistance" (U.S. Department of Education, n.d.).

Here's Information Regarding Section 504 of the Rehabilitation Act (1998)

The Rehabilitation Act defines an individual with a disability as one who:

- has a physical or mental impairment which substantially limits one or more of such person's major life activities
- has a record of such an impairment
- is regarded as having such an impairment

Section 504 federal regulations require a school district to provide FAPE to each qualified student with a disability who is in the school district's jurisdiction, regardless of the nature or severity of the disability. Under Section 504, FAPE consists of the provision of regular or special education to meet the student's individual educational needs as adequately as the needs of nondisabled students. Students with a physical or mental impairment that substantially restricts one or more major life activities are eligible for services under Section 504. Some schools use Section 504 to support students with learning disabilities (LD) who need instructional accommodations rather than the specially designed instruction provided under IDEA.

Here's Information Regarding Americans With Disabilities Act (ADA) and Americans With Disabilities Amendments Act of 2008 (ADAA)

Because the Rehabilitation Act of 1973 preceded the enactment of the ADA by nearly 20 years, Section 504 of the Rehabilitation Act has generally been the basis for disabilities protection in the nation's public schools.

The ADA, passed in 1990, was the first comprehensive civil rights law for people with disabilities. It applied to all state and local government programs, including public schools, and all places of public accommodation, including non-religiously controlled colleges and universities and test agencies.

ADAA 2008 was passed by Congress in 2008 and became effective on January 1, 2009, amending the ADA. It also includes an amendment to the Rehabilitation Act of 1973 (Rehabilitation Act) that affects the meaning of disability in Section 504.

According to the NCLD, the ADAA continues to include all public and private institutions listed earlier. It also continues to define an individual with a disability as one with a physical or mental impairment that substantially limits one or more major life activities, including learning disabilities (NCLD, 2009).

Before ADAA, the definition of major life activities included but was not limited to the following: caring for oneself, performing manual tasks, seeing, hearing, speaking, breathing, learning, and working. The following activities have been added: eating, sleeping, walking, standing, lifting, bending, reading, concentrating, thinking, and communicating. In addition, the legislation clarified that an impairment substantially limiting one major life activity does not need to limit other life activities to be considered a disability.

Before ADAA, several Supreme Court cases established that the decision of whether an individual has a disability under the ADA must take into account the effects, both positive and negative, of any mitigating measures used by that individual. This would include whether a student was on medication and the effects of the medication on the disability, assistive technology used, medical supplies, and so on. ADAA now requires the "substantially limits" decision to be made without regard to any impact of mitigating measures. For example, schools can no longer consider the effect of medication on a student with attention disorders including inattention, hyperactivity, and/or impulsivity (attention deficit disorder/attention deficit hyperactivity disorder [ADD/ADHD]), asthma, diabetes, and so on. In addition, the ADAA provides an expansive list of mitigating measures. Such measures include but are not limited to the following: medication, medical supplies, equipment or appliances, low-vision devices (except eyeglasses or contact lenses), hearing aids, cochlear implants, assistive technology, learned behavioral or adaptive neurological modifications, and reasonable accommodations.

According to Kaloi and Stanberry (2009), there are several situations where eligibility for Section 504 should now be reconsidered since the revisions in ADAA. Among them are:

- When a student has been evaluated for eligibility under IDEA and found to be ineligible
- When a student previously eligible for and receiving services under IDEA is determined to no longer need special education services
- When a student is determined to have a disability but only needs accommodations and not specific special services

Here Are Some Important 504 Accommodations for Students With Language-Based Learning Disabilities

The following list provides some reasonable accommodations under Section 504. The list has been adapted from a list provided by the NCLD. This list has been condensed and modified specifically to those with language-based learning disabilities (LD OnLine, 2011).

Classroom Environment and Seating

- Preferential seating (close to where the teacher teaches, away from auditory and visual distractions, near a peer who can offer assistance, increased distance between desks)
- Classroom has predictable daily routines with schedule changes discussed before they occur
- Short concentrated periods or work with breaks
- Small group instruction
- Identify teaching style/student match (e.g., structured, nurturing, etc.)

Assignments and Homework

- Allow extra time to complete assigned work.
- Shorten assignments/work periods.
- Simplify complex directions.
- Repeat oral instructions.
- Gain the student's attention before giving oral instructions.
- Pair written instructions with oral instructions.
- Develop private signal from pupil to teacher to request repetition of oral directions.
- Reduce amount of homework to a specified amount of time or assignments per night.
- Permit assignments to be printed or typewritten without penalty.
- Permit writing assignments to be completed with computer-aided technology.
- Permit resubmitted assignments.
- Do not grade handwriting or spelling (if not a spelling test).

Test Taking and Grading

- Provide written outline of main points and supporting details prior to tests.
- Allow open-book exams.
- Allow outline or notes during exams.
- Give exams orally.
- Give take-home tests.
- Allow the student to dictate answers to an audio recorder or an adult.
- Give frequent short quizzes rather than long exams.
- Allow extra time for exams.
- Allow tests to be taken untimed with specified short breaks.
- Read test item to the student.

Home/School/Community Communication

- Increased frequency of parent/teacher/student interaction to a specified frequency
- Increased frequency of reporting progress

Aids and Technology

- Provide audio room systems to increase the teacher's voice over background distractions.
- Provide keyboarding skills training.
- Provide a computer with appropriate software for written assignments or in-class note taking.
- Provide textbooks through ebook or on audio download.
- Provide an extra set of textbooks to have at home if ebook is not available.

Learning Strategies

- Provide auditory and written directions at the same time.
- Use consistent graphic organizers (webs, Venn diagrams, Cornell notes, T charts, etc.).
- Encourage (multicolored) outlining/underlining when reading.
- Use tactile and manipulative aids in teaching.
- Provide written outline of lesson or written notes of lecture material.
- Write main points of the lesson on the board.
- Permit devices that will record classroom lectures.
- Avoid oral reading (especially important for students with a word-finding disorder).
- Encourage oral reading.
- Teach phonetic decoding skills.
- Use guided reading, echo reading, paired reading, or simultaneous reading approach to reading acquisition.
- Teach auditory discrimination skills to reading acquisition.
- Teach underlining strategies.
- Teach skills to obtain the main idea and supporting details.
- Use graphic organizers with literature to increase understanding of characters, setting, plot, conflict, conflict resolution, conclusion.

Written Expression

- Provide instruction in brainstorming, outlining, and use of webs for organization.
- Provide specialized software for word processing.
- Provide homework assignments or teacher's notes online or handed to the student so that the student does not need to copy from board or book.

Spelling

- Use an electronic spell checker (handheld and/or computer).
- Do not grade spelling on assignments other than spelling.
- Limit spelling list words.
- Circle the correct version of a word given several choices for testing.

Math

- Permit use of calculators.
- Provide graph paper to space numbers.
- Teach strategies to increase success with math facts or computation.
- Provide worksheets or workbooks with space to complete the work.
- Provide access to math book and math workbook online for homework and additional practice.

Organization and Planning

- Use online assignment listings.
- Provide the student with assignment book.
- Check that homework assignments are written in full detail.
- Provide a written checklist for getting organized.
- Provide a notebook with dividers and folders for work.
- Check the desk/notebook for neatness and appropriate organization.

This is not an inclusive list of accommodations that can be offered under a Section 504 plan. I tried to list the ones that would be most beneficial to a student with a language-based learning disability.

Here Are the Agencies That Enforce the Laws

Two groups in the U.S. Department of Education are designed to oversee and enforce the laws that are the overriding umbrella by which educational services are provided. This is broken down by state as well through state educational agencies.

Office for Civil Rights (OCR)

OCR, an office of the U.S. Department of Education, enforces the ADAA and the Rehabilitation Act, including Section 504.

The Office of Special Education and Rehabilitative Services (OSERS)

OSERS, also a division of the U.S. Department of Education, administers IDEA.

State Educational Agencies

Each state educational agency is responsible for administering IDEA within the state and distributing the funds for special education programs.

Conclusion

This chapter provides the groundwork for understanding students with language-based learning disabilities. Definitions are provided to better understand learning disabilities overall as well as the acronyms used throughout all educational environments. It provides information regarding the public laws that regulate how students with disabilities are educated.

Lastly, just as this chapter began, I want to encourage all of us to imagine what students who struggle and have a learning disability face each day. As adults, we must always focus on how our actions, both verbal and nonverbal, affect those who receive our services. As we all know, if a person does not think that potential is limited, then this person strives to reach his or her fullest potential. Here are a few reminders as we begin the journey into this text regarding language-based learning disabilities and as we go forth to provide the best strategies, attitudes, and skills to assist students.

- Focus on student strengths, talents, and accomplishments.
- Provide opportunities for students to display responsibility and/or leadership role.
- Make time to talk alone with each student.
- Look for the accomplishments of each student.
- Send positive notes home.
- Avoid using a child as a negative example to others.
- Avoid questioning a child's motivation or effort.
- Assist students with strategies that will better measure their knowledge.
- Assist students with strategies for developing skills.

We can be key team members in assisting students who are struggling and those with learning disabilities maximize their potential. Imagine, for our students, everyday success in the learning environment.

References

American Speech-Language-Hearing Association. (n.d.). *Language-based learning disabilities.* Retrieved December 28, 2009, from http://www.asha.org

Cohen, M. (2007, July 8). AD/HD under IDEA. *Child advocate—helping parents and professionals.* Retrieved December 28, 2009, from http://www.childadvocate.net

Dockrell, J., Messer, D., George, R., & Easton, S. (1998). Children with word finding difficulties: Prevalence, presentation, and naming problems. *International Journal of Language and Communication Disorders, 13*(2), 125–142.

German, D. (1998, February 1). *Prevalence estimates for word finding difficulties in LD students: Implications for assessment and instructional accommodations.* Lecture conducted from the Learning Disabilities Association, Washington, DC.

Kaloi, L., & Stanberry, K. (2009, March 12). *Section 504 in 2009: Broader eligibility, more accommodations.* Retrieved February 6, 2011, from http://www.ncld.org

LD OnLine. (2011, March 22). *LD Basics: Learning disability fast fact.* Retrieved February 5, 2011, from http://www.ldonline.org

LD OnLine. (n.d.). *LD basics: What is a learning disability?* Retrieved February 5, 2011, from http://www.ldonline.org

Lewis, B. (2007, October). Literacy problems associated with childhood apraxia of speech. *Language, Learning, and Education,* 10–16.

National Center for Learning Disabilities. (2009, March 12). *Americans with Disabilities Amendments Act (ADAA).* Retrieved February 6, 2011, from http://www.ncld.org

National Center for Learning Disabilities. (n.d.). *Laws protecting students. Learning disabilities.* Retrieved February 5, 2011, from http://www.ncld.org

National Center for Learning Disabilities. (2009, March 26). *LD checklist of signs and symptoms.* Retrieved February 5, 2011, from http://ncld.org

National Institutes of Health. (2010, October 18). *NINDS learning disorder information page.* Retrieved February 5, 2011, from http://www.ninds.nih.gov/disorders/learningdisabilities/learningdisabilities.htm

Reed, V. (2005). *An introduction to children with language disorders* (3rd ed.). Boston, MA: Pearson/Allyn and Bacon.

Sharma, R., Purdy, S., & Kelly, A. (2009). Comorbidity of auditory processing, language, and reading disorders. *Journal of Speech, Language, and Hearing Research, 52,* 706–722.

Sousa, D. A. (2007). *How the special needs brain learns* (2nd ed.). Thousand Oaks, CA: Corwin Press.

U.S. Department of Education. (n.d.). *Protecting students with disabilities: Frequently asked questions about Section 504 and the education of children with disabilities.* Retrieved February 6, 2011, from http://www.ed.gov

U.S. Department of Education. (2008, January 2). *The Elementary and Secondary School Act.* Retrieved February 6, 2011, from http://www.ed.gov

U.S. Department of Education. (2008, February). *Lead & manage my school: The Individuals with Disabilities Education Act (IDEA): Provisions related to children with disabilities enrolled by their parents in private schools.* Retrieved February 6, 2011, from http://www.ed.gov

2

Diagnostics

Introduction

With Response to Intervention (RTI), students should receive differentiated instruction within their classroom (Tier I Intervention) and in small groups (Tier 2 Intervention) before a more individualized and intensive plan is initiated (Tier 3 Intervention). When a student is referred for Tier 3 intervention, evaluations may be indicated for special education services. In a private setting, these referrals for evaluations may occur while a student is in any tier of RTI or may be struggling within the curriculum and not identified through the RTI process.

It is the position of the American Speech-Language-Hearing Association (ASHA) that speech-language pathologists play a critical and direct role in the development of literacy for children and adolescents with communication disorders. As with receptive and expressive language development, the same components of language—phonology, morphology, syntax, semantics, and pragmatics—play a vital role in reading and writing (Wolf Nelson et al., 2001). A student also must be able to participate fully in a classroom environment in order to gain academic knowledge. Full participation for academic success includes other areas such as following classroom directions, retrieving information quickly and accurately, auditory and reading comprehension, written language expression, the ability to reason through a situation, as well as many other areas that speech-language pathologists typically assess. The speech-language pathologist's involvement with literacy and learning skills may start with a universal screening as part of an RTI process, involvement with strategies through RTI, or a comprehensive evaluation that assesses the language components that may be affecting these skills.

For young children, deficits in areas such as morphological and phonological awareness, auditory short-term memory, word-finding skills, and sequencing provide us with insight as areas to monitor for literacy and learning success. For elementary students, assessing components of language such as morphology, phonology, syntax, and semantics provides information and direction for assisting students who are struggling with literacy and learning. When the students are older (fourth grade through high school), I often state that I am looking for a needle in a haystack. What is noted with these students is that they are very bright and have learned strategies to perform fairly well in school. At about the fourth grade, when the academic subjects become increasingly complex and increased critical thinking is required, the strategies that the students are using are no longer adequate. Parents of these students often report that they have always seen areas of concern, but as long as they (the parents) assist with homework each night, their student does well in school. Also, the parents begin to realize that by the fourth grade or so their student should be more independent with his or her homework; however, they are not seeing signs of moving in that direction. In order to determine the appropriate strategies for a student, the speech-language pathologist may need to complete an evaluation that will assist in determining why the student is having academic difficulty and if there is an underlying speech or language disorder.

Preschool/Kindergarten Children

The signs that there are potential language-based learning difficulties usually appear by prekindergarten or kindergarten. For example, parents often will report that their student would appear to know a letter, sound, or word one day but not the next, which could be indicative of a word-finding disorder. Prekindergarten teachers often will determine that a student is struggling with phonological awareness activities such as rhyming and determining words in sentences, syllables in words, and sounds in words. Parents may report that their child has difficulty following directions.

Several language milestones may indicate that a student may be at risk for ongoing learning difficulties. The student may have difficulty:

- using verb tenses such as present progressive and past tense
- using the plural form of the verb
- communicating, owing to decreased receptive and expressive vocabulary skills
- performing tasks that require auditory short-term memory such as:
  - following increasingly complex directions
  - repeating words (items needed from the store) or sentences verbatim (What did I ask you to do?)
  - remembering and repeating verses in a book, poem, or song
- perceiving sounds in words correctly
- understanding and using rhyming words
- naming tasks rapidly and automatically
- repeating words with discrimination errors
- answering "why" and "how come" questions (beginning critical thinking skills)

Although tests for younger children may not specify the significance of the test item on specific learning skills, one can make informed clinical decisions regarding the implications of the test results and the potential for learning difficulties by understanding the underlying language area that the item is testing.

Morphology Introduction

Nunes, Bryant, and Bindman (2006) found that morphological awareness has a significant impact on reading in the early years. Morphological awareness can be defined as understanding the structure and form of a given word. These include structures such as present progressive (verb of to be + -ing), plurals /s/ and /z/, past tense /d/ and /t/, third person singular /s/ and /z/, comparative and superlatives /er/ and /est/.

Phonology Introduction

Torgesen, Wagner, and Rashotte (1997) reported that children who began first grade with phonological awareness skills below the 20th percentile lagged behind their peers in word identification and word decoding throughout elementary school. Phonological awareness skills during the preschool years include skills such as understanding that words are composed of segments of sounds (phonemic awareness); understanding and producing rhyming words; segmenting compound words; and identifying the beginning, middle, and ending sounds in words.

Auditory Short-Term Memory Skills Introduction

Children with receptive and expressive specific language impairment perform significantly poorer than their peers on auditory short-term memory tasks (Nickisch & Kries, 2009). Auditory short-term memory can be defined as the ability to remember what one hears for a short amount of time. Typically, this is seconds. Difficulty with auditory short-term memory will have a significant impact once the child enters school. Short-term auditory memory can be assessed for young children with any testing item that asks the child to repeat a sentence or series of words or numbers verbatim or having the child follow oral directions with increasing complexity and length.

Word Finding Introduction

Adults often state, "It is on the tip of my tongue." Children often look to their parents for help when they are trying to retrieve information that is well known to them, but they are unable to retrieve it to express their thoughts. Preschool and kindergarten children with word-finding difficulties may demonstrate expressive difficulties that can be observed with expressing colors, shapes, letters, or familiar objects or generating a list of items in a category.

Possible Assessment Tools

The following provides a list of assessment tools that may be used when evaluating a preschool- or kindergarten-age child. Any of these tests could be used during the universal screenings provided as part of the RTI process or could be used collectively for a broader view of language skills. Some of these instruments may not specifically state that the items in the test measure morphology, phonology, semantics, syntax, pragmatics, or word finding. The examiner will be able to assess specific testing items that do indeed measure these language areas.

- Clinical Evaluation of Language Fundamentals—Preschool: This tool includes nine subtests: Sentence and Word Structure, Expressive Vocabulary, Concepts, Following Directions, Recalling Sentences, Basic Concepts, Word Classes, and Phonological Awareness. It is standardized for children ages 3 through 6 years (Semel, Wiig, & Secord, 2004).

- Test of Examining Expressive Morphology: This test examines the following areas: present progressive, third-person singular, and past tense verbs; plural and possessive nouns; derived adjectives; and irregular comparative and superlative adjectives. It is standardized for children ages 3 to 7 (Shipley, Stone, & Sue, 1983).

- Dynamic Screening for Phonological Awareness (DSPA): The DSPA is a 20-item screening for sound and syllable deletion as an indicator for literacy success. It is norm referenced for children ages 4 through 6 years (Sittner Bridges & Catts, 2011).

- Phonological Awareness and Literacy Screening: This prekindergarten screening targets beginning sounds, blending, rhyming, and sound-to-letter segmentation (Invernizzi, 2004).

- Phonological Awareness Profile: This is a criterion-referenced profile for children ages 5 through 8 years. It measures rhyming, segmenting, isolation, deletion, substitution, and blending. It also includes subtests for phoneme/grapheme correspondence, decoding, and invented spelling (Roberston & Salter, 1995).

- Phonological Awareness Test 2 (PAT 2): The PAT 2 is norm referenced for children beginning at age 5 years. This test measures identification of phonemes by word position, manipulating root words, syllables and phonemes, phoneme isolation, and sound/symbol relationship (Robertson & Salter, 2007).

- Preschool Language Scale 4 (PLS 4): This scale includes auditory comprehension and language expression items for children from birth to 6 years 11 months. There are many individual items on the scale that assess morphology and phonology (Zimmerman, Steiner, & Pond, 2002).

- Preschool Language Scale 5 (PLS 5): This scale is due out in spring 2011. Information regarding the scale states that there are more items to assess for early literacy and phonological awareness skills (Zimmerman, Steiner, & Pond, 2011).

- Preschool Language Scale 4 Screening Test (PLS 4 Screening Test): This test identifies the abilities of children who are at risk for a language disorder and need further evaluation (Zimmerman, Steiner, & Pond, 2005).

- Test of Word Finding: This test is designed to use with children as young as 4 years 0 months. It offers four different naming tasks to assess for word finding. These include picture naming for nouns and verbs, sentence completion naming, and picture naming categories (German, 2000).

In conclusion, the speech-language pathologist can begin to identify areas that may have an academic impact on young children in preschool and kindergarten. As stated previously, difficulty in learning to read and write can involve any of the components of language—phonology, morphology, syntax, semantics, and pragmatics. Academic success also is based on the ability to follow classroom directions, use reasoning skills for understanding classroom information, and recall information quickly and accurately to communicate and learn effectively.

School-Age Assessment Essentials Introduction

For the school-age student, a comprehensive evaluation, in addition to results of screenings, progress monitoring from an RTI process, and reports from teachers and parents, may be indicated. The evaluation should include reports or rating scales from educators and parents, a measure of receptive and expressive vocabulary, receptive and expressive language, and word finding, at the least. Additional tests that specifically address skills in silent and oral reading fluency, written expression, or a more in-depth assessment of phonological awareness skills or reasoning skills may be warranted.

Rating Scales

Parents, teachers, and older students can provide valuable insight to the areas that are most difficult for the student. This information can assist in directing the areas that should be assessed during the evaluation.

- Clinical Evaluation of Language Function Observational Rating Scale: This scale provides a view of the student's skills in the areas of listening, speaking, reading, and writing. The examiner should consider any area that is rated as occurring as often or always to be areas of concern. The examiner can use these rated areas to assist in determining the critical areas that require further assessment (Semel, Wiig, & Secord, 1995).

- Fisher's Auditory Checklist: This checklist provides statements that could be indicative of a language or auditory processing disorder. Questions include statements regarding listening to directions, following auditory directions, sound discrimination, and difficulty with phonics. It also includes short-term auditory memory statements such as recalling a sequence that is heard or recalling other auditory information (Fisher, 1985).

This checklist is designed to determine when to refer a student to an audiologist for central auditory processing testing. This checklist also could be used by the speech-language pathologist to determine if further evaluation for receptive and expressive language skills is required (Fisher, 1985).

Receptive and Expressive Vocabulary Measures

Receptive and expressive vocabulary knowledge provides greater information than just current vocabulary skills. The student must demonstrate semantic knowledge of vocabulary for a specific subject for success in that subject. For example, while working with a student prepare for a fifth-grade science test regarding the solar system, I asked the student which planet had craters. We had already discussed that there is no air or water on Mars; therefore, there could be no life. The student seemed confused, so in my speech therapy mode of thinking of whether this could be a vocabulary issue, I asked the student to define craters. He defined craters as tiny animals. It was then obvious that he had missed or misunderstood a third-grade science vocabulary word of craters and thought that craters were actually creatures! Then we worked on reasoning skills! If there is no air and no water, could there be creatures on Mars?

Secondly, a statistically significant discrepancy between receptive and expressive vocabulary scores provides information regarding possible word-finding difficulties. The examiner is always encouraged to write down all responses that the student gives. This includes the first response, self-corrections, definitions, fillers (um, you know), gestures, and delays in response time. This comparison also can provide information regarding attention and focus as well as word finding.

Receptive and expressive vocabulary measures include:

- Comprehensive Receptive and Expressive Vocabulary Test II (Wallace & Hammill, 2008)

- Expressive One Word Picture Vocabulary Test (Brownell, 2011)

- Expressive Vocabulary Test 2 (Williams, 2007)

- Peabody Picture Vocabulary Test 4 (Dunn & Dunn, 2007)

- Receptive One Word Picture Vocabulary Test (Brownell, 2011)

By documenting the responses during the expressive vocabulary test, the examiner is able to gain a broader view of a student's knowledge and retrieval.

Word-Finding Measures

Diane German (2000) identifies six groups of children who would benefit from a word-finding assessment. These include children with learning disabilities, language disorders, specific language impairment, fluency disorders, known brain pathologies, and attention deficit/hyperactivity disorders. Dr. German provides response categories for analysis in the Test of Word Finding II. These include semantically, phonemically, and perceptual substitutions (German, 2000, pp. 45–46).

Semantically related categories include naming the class in which a word belongs; substituting words from the same word class; and using a subgroup of the word by telling its function, location, or from what it is made. It also includes words that are associated with the target word.

Phonemically related substitutions include exchanging, substituting, adding, or omitting sounds or words. It also includes substituting a similar word (octagon for octopus) or using a rhyming response.

Perceptual substitutions include visual misperceptions (horse for dog) or only visualizing part of the picture (horse for statue).

Dr. German (2009) identifies three patterns of errors. These include:

- Pattern 1: "Slip of the Tongue" error. This type of error may indicate a failure to access the word's semantic or syntactic features.

- Pattern 2: "Tip of the Tongue" error. This type of error results in a failure to access any of the word's form information.

- Pattern 3: "Twist of the Tongue" error: This type of error results in an incomplete access to the word's form, syllabic frame, or segmental sound content.

Word-finding measures include:

- Test of Word Finding II (German, 2000)

- Test of Adolescent/Adult Word Finding (German, 1990)

- Test of Word Finding in Discourse (German, 1991)

Receptive and Expressive Language Testing

The speech-language pathologist also needs to assess overall receptive and expressive language skills. Regardless of the standardized measure used, the speech-language pathologist must determine how the performance and results relate to academic areas and the possible outcome of deficits in specific areas. The following tests as well as others that are familiar to the examiner should be considered.

Receptive and expressive language measures include:

- Clinical Evaluation of Language Fundamentals, 4th Edition: This test determines the nature of the language disorder. Supplemental subtests include Phonological Awareness, Rapid Automatic Naming, Digit Span, Sequences, Word Associations, and Memory. It also includes the Observational Rating Scale discussed previously in this chapter in addition to a pragmatic profile (Semel, Wiig, & Secord, 2003).

- Comprehensive Assessment of Spoken Language: This test assesses the following language components: lexical/semantic, syntax, supralinguistics, and pragmatic skills (Carrow-Woolfolk, 1999).

- Test of Adolescent and Adult Language, 4th Edition: This test measures spoken and written language. It includes measures for word opposites, derivations and similarities, spoken analogies, sentence combination, and orthographic use (Hammill, Brown, Larsen, & Wiederholt, 2007).

- Test of Auditory Processing 2 (TAPS 2): This test measures phonological awareness, auditory short-term memory, auditory comprehension, and reasoning (Martin & Brownell, 2005).

- Test of Language Developmental—Intermediate, 4th Edition: This test measures semantics (i.e., meaning and thought) and grammar (i.e., syntax and morphology) skills and listening, organizing, and measuring speaking abilities (Hammill & Newcomer, 2008).

- Test of Oral and Written Language Scales (OWLS): These scales provide a measure that assesses many areas that are important for academic success. This includes multiple word meanings, logic, figurative language, inferences, and sentence formation (Carrow-Woolfolk, 1996).

It is vital to use the latest edition of a test in order to obtain the most reliable results; therefore, speech-language pathologists should use the preceding information as a guide and always check for the latest version before a test is used. It also is important to choose one that will assist the examiner in formulating the plan for therapy that will impact academic success. If a test that is given does not indicate an underlying receptive or expressive language disorder to the learning difficulties, it does not mean that a language disorder does not exist. The problem areas may be identified better through another test.

Another option is to gather and analyze a language sample. Pamela Hadley (1998) provides two different protocols for eliciting language samples in school-age children. The first is gathering a sample in an interview format. The second provides a sampling during a narrative. Schmidek (1997) provides information on gathering, transcribing, segmenting, marking, and analyzing narrative samples.

Central Auditory Processing Disorder (C)APD

A simplistic definition of central auditory processing refers to the efficiency and effectiveness by which the central nervous system uses auditory information (Bellis et al., 2005). Many professionals include phonological awareness, attention to memory for auditory information, comprehension, and interpretation of auditorily presented information. Although there may be a comorbid language disorder that would include these areas, these are not truly auditory processing. According to ASHA (C)APD technical report, (C)APD may lead to, coexist, or be associated with difficulties in higher order language, learning, and communication function (Bellis et al., 2005). (C)APD can lead to or be associated with difficulties in learning, speech, and/or language (including written language involving reading and spelling). Owing to the possibility of comorbid speech, language, and/or learning disorders, students with suspected (C)APD should have a multidisciplinary evaluation. The audiologist will assess the following:

- Auditory discrimination: The ability to differentiate similar acoustic stimuli that differ in frequency, intensity, and/or temporal parameters

- Auditory temporal processing and patterning tests: The ability to analyze acoustic events over time

- Dichotic speech tests: The ability to separate or integrate auditory stimuli presented to each ear simultaneously

- Monaural speech tests: The ability to recognize speech stimuli presented one ear at a time

- Binaural speech tests: The ability to process intensity or time difference of acoustic stimuli

- Electroacoustic and electrophysiological measures: Recording of acoustic signals and electrical potentials of activities generated by the central nervous system (Bellis et al., 2005)

Results of the testing completed by the audiologist will provide valuable information as to how a student may perform in a classroom. This student may benefit from a frequency modulation (FM) system in the classroom in order to perceive more accurately what the teacher is saying. The audiologist can provide invaluable insight as to the particular way a child processes auditory information. This information can assist in determining how this will impact a student's ability to process auditory information in the classroom and accommodations or modifications that may need to be in place for optimal learning.

The speech-language pathologist should assess the language difficulties that also may be present. This may include completion of rating scales of listening behaviors, classroom observations as well as a full speech and/or language testing that should include receptive and expressive vocabulary and language, and word finding. Speech-language pathologists use the following tests for screening:

- SCAN 3C: This screening and diagnostic tool is designed for children ages 5 years to 12 years 11 months. The screening tool provides the following assessments:
  - Gap Detection: Assesses the presence of a temporal processing problem that may influence the ability to comprehend running speech
  - Auditory Figure Ground: Tests the child's ability to listen with background noise
  - Competing Words (Free Recall): Dichotic listening task

  Diagnostic tests include:
  - Filtered Words: Indicates ability to process speech when the signal is distorted or compromised by a poor acoustic environment
  - Competing Words: Dichotic listening task
  - Competing Sentences: Provides information about the maturation of the auditory nervous system (Keith, 2009)

- SCAN 3 A: This screening and diagnostic test is designed for persons 13 years to 50 years 11 months of age. It provides the following subtests:
  - Gap Detection: Assesses temporal processing problems
  - Auditory Figure Ground (+0 dB): Tests ability to listen with background noise
  - Competing Words (Free Recall): Dichotic listening task

  Diagnostic tests include:
  - Filtered Words: Indicates ability to process speech when the signal is distorted or compromised by a poor acoustic environment
  - Competing Words (Directed Ear): Dichotic listening task
  - Competing Sentences: Provides information about the maturation of the nervous system

  Supplementary tests include:
  - Auditory Figure Ground
  - Time Compressed Sentence (Keith, 2009)

- Differential Screening Test for Processing (DSTP): This screening is designed for children ages 6 years to 12 years. The purpose of this test is to differentiate among the various levels of auditory and language processing. It also identifies areas for referral or further evaluation. The three levels of processing are acoustic, acoustic-linguistic, and linguistic (Richard & Ferre, 2006).

If the student is struggling academically, the multidisciplinary assessment also may include a psychometric evaluation to assess intelligence, achievement, attention issues, or other areas that are relevant for academic success.

In summary, testing for language disorders that may affect learning should include at least a measure of receptive and expressive vocabulary and language (including morphology, phonology, syntax, semantics, pragmatics, auditory short-term memory, reasoning, and word finding). Referral to an audiologist also is suggested if a (C)APD is suspected. Speech-language pathologists are encouraged strongly to use their clinical judgment and expertise to describe what is observed during testing. If the speech-language pathologist considers only the total standard score, the problem area may not be properly identified. This may lead to continued academic problems versus remediating the specific area that is causing the learning difficulty.

Many other tests can be used as part of the assessment. These include tests for oral and silent reading, assessment of written expression, phonological awareness, or problem solving.

Written Language Expression

Students with language disorders typically demonstrate difficulty in written language expression. The following written language expression tests are available to assess this area:

- OWLS: Written portion provides an assessment of written language expression for students 5 years to 21 years 11 months and includes written language conventions, linguistic concepts, sentence combinations, and metalinguistic use (Carrow-Woolfolk, 1996).

- Test of Written Language, 4th Edition (TOWL 4): This test is norm referenced for students ages 9 years 0 months to 17 years 11 months. It measures conventional, linguistic, and conceptual aspects of students' writing, which includes mechanics, vocabulary, syntax, grammar, plot, and character development (Hammill, Brown, & Larsen, 2009).

- Test of Early Written Language 2 (TEWL 2): This test is standardized for students ages 4 years 0 months to 10 years 11 months and measures basic and contextual writing through spelling, linguistic and metalinguistic use, and sentence combination (Herron, Hresko, & Peak, 2001).

- Woodcock-Johnson II: This test offers a written language subtest. It measures spelling, writing fluency, and editing through writing samples (Woodcock, McGrew, & Mather, 2001).

- Wechsler Individual Achievement Test III: This test is standardized for persons 4 years to almost 60 years of age. It measures alphabetic writing; word fluency; sentence and paragraph writing including mechanics, organization, and vocabulary; as well as essay writing including mechanics, organization, theme development, and vocabulary (Wechsler, 2009).

When choosing a test for written language, make sure it assesses the areas that are most pertinent for a student. For example, a student with a word-finding disorder may write grammatically correct sentences, but they may be very basic. Tests for written language may not assess the student's ability to use synonyms of words or sentences with significant description (adjectives, adverbs, phrases) or the ability to write compound or complex sentences.

Phonological Awareness Assessment

Phonological awareness is defined as the explicit understanding of a word's sound structure. This includes the ability to segment words into syllables, identify and produce rhyming words, identify individual sounds in words, blend sounds to make words, and segment words into individual sounds (Gillon, 2002). If the speech-language pathologist determines that phonological awareness is an area that is significantly impacting academic success, one may consider a deeper assessment than what may be provided as a subsection of another test. These are:

- Phonological Awareness Test 2: This test is standardized for students ages 5 to 9 and provides an assessment into every area that is important to be a good phonics reader. This includes: rhyming, segmentation, isolation and substitutions with manipulatives, blending, graphemes, decoding, and invented spelling (Robertson & Salter, 2007).

- Comprehensive Test of Phonological Processing: This measure is standardized for students from 5 years to 24 years 11 months and measures the following areas: phonological, phonological memory, and rapid naming (Wagner, Torgesen, & Rashotte, 1999).

- Test of Phonological Awareness, 2nd Edition: This test is standardized for students ages 5 years 0 months to 8 years 0 months and is designed to administer to an entire class. It measures the following:
  - Kindergarten: Same sound and different sound at the beginning of words
  - First grade: Same sound and different sound at the end of the words (Torgesen & Bryant, 2004)

Problem Solving

The ability to problem solve is key. A student must be able to think critically about the information that is learned. This means applying what is learned to what the student already knows as well as being able to relate information to other circumstances. This is where true learning occurs. The following tests provide in-depth assessment of problem-solving skills:

- Test of Problem Solving 3 (TOPS 3): This test provides a more comprehensive assessment for students ages 6 through 12 regarding the ability to make inferences, understanding negative questions, making predictions, sequencing, problem solving, and determining the cause (Bowers, Huisingh, & LoGiudice, 2005).

- Test of Problem Solving 2 (TOPS 2): TOPS 2 for adolescents ages 12 through 17 measures the following areas: making inferences, determining solutions, problem solving, interpreting perspectives, and transferring insight (Bowers, Huisingh, & LoGiudice, 2004).

Determining the Significance of the Testing Results

All of the classroom observations, progress monitoring, rating scales, and comprehensive testing have been completed. What is the next step? The speech-language pathologist needs to put a picture together of what the results mean. Where is the needle in the haystack? I find it most useful to examine the subtest standard scores in comparison to other subtest scores on the measure if there is more than one subtest. For tests that provide one overall standard score such as a vocabulary test, I compare the receptive vocabulary test with the expressive vocabulary test. Subtest scores or comparison of similar tests provides the means of finding the possible area or areas that are causing academic concerns. Keep in mind that it is often subtest areas that may be causing academic difficulties instead of a total score on the test.

Possible Profiles

- Decreased receptive and/or expressive vocabulary skills: This would be observed in difficulty with subject-based vocabulary. The student may learn the vocabulary words expected in a current textbook chapter but may not have learned the vocabulary for the same subject area that was introduced in earlier grade levels. This will affect the students comprehension of the current material presented.

- Gap between receptive and expressive vocabulary: The receptive and expressive vocabulary scores should be used for comparison. If the receptive score is statistically higher than the expressive score, this student should be further examined for word-finding difficulties, which would need to be assessed further. Again, the examiner should document the responses obtained during the expressive vocabulary measure in order to determine whether the gap exists because of decreased expressive vocabulary or a profile that is indicative of a word-finding disorder. This gap may exist only if the examiner scores the first response as incorrect. If the student produces an incorrect response initially but then self-corrects, the examiner knows that the student knows the vocabulary. If the second response is scored then the examiner may miss the gap that would indicate a word-finding disorder. I always qualify when I report the results that the student's initial response was used in scoring the test.

  If the expressive score is statistically higher than the receptive score and other inconsistent response patterns are present throughout testing, the student may need further assessment by a child psychologist or other disciplines that specialize in attention and focus issues.

- Decreased receptive or expressive language scores: Again it is important to review the specific response pattern regardless of the standard scores obtained. The student may demonstrate difficulties in the areas of phonology, morphology, syntax, semantics, or pragmatics that will have an impact on academic success.

- Decreased word-finding skills: The ability to quickly and accurately retrieve information will impact oral reading accuracy, classroom participation, written expression, and test-taking skills.

- Decreased auditory short-term memory: Difficulty with auditory short-term memory will hinder a student in following classroom directions, remembering sentences for dictation on spelling tests, and/or following classroom lectures.

In conclusion, a comprehensive language evaluation of a student experiencing academic difficulties is crucial. The speech-language pathologist is encouraged to judge individual subtest performance critically and not just overall standard scores. With appropriate remediation of specific deficit areas, the student can then be successful in all subject matters where this deficiency has presented a problem. From the speech-language pathologist working only with preschoolers to those working with students through high school, an understanding of how speech and language disorders affect academic success could make a difference in students' daily performance, passing statewide testing, having acceptable scores of college entrance exams, or going to a trade school or junior college or setting their sights on the career of their dreams. We often hold the key to academic success. The first step is to identify where the disorder lies.

What Happens After the Evaluation

After the evaluation is completed, the speech-language pathologist needs to report the results in a format that other professionals can review as well as one that is parent friendly. One report that serves both purposes is often difficult. I have found that one report format can be used if I provide a description of the test, specific examples of my observations during testing, as well as specific examples of how the student performed. I also encourage parents to sit in on the evaluation so that they can observe how their child is performing on the test. This makes the conversation regarding the results easier because specific examples from the evaluation can be presented.

In the written report, I state what standard scores are considered within the average range. I also provide a graph where I document the student's standard score on each subtest. This provides the parents with a visual means of understanding standard scores and gaps between scores. The following graph provides an adequate representation of the standard scores that may be reported (Table 2–1).

Form 2–1 shows the format that I present while providing written results of an evaluation. As stated previously this format provides a description of what the test measured as well as specific testing results and examples.

Table 2–1. Graph of Standard Scores

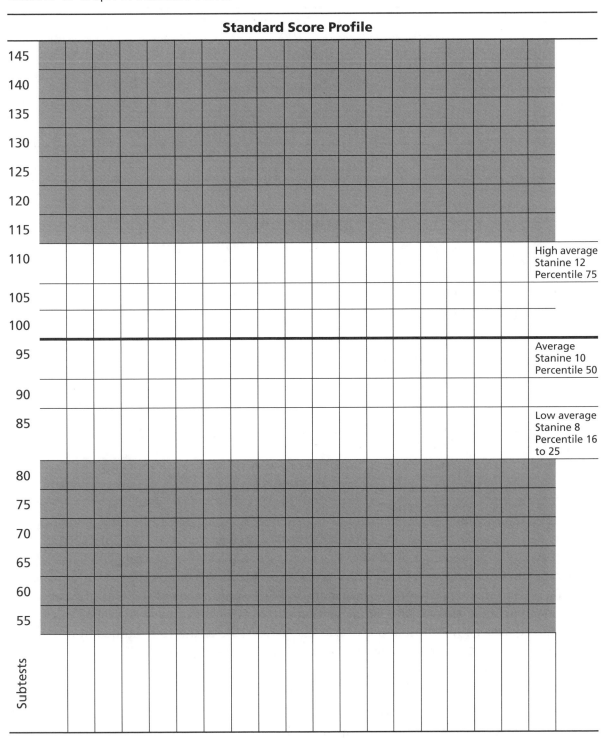

Note: Developed by Margo Kinzer Courter, MBA, MA, CCC-SLP.

■ Form 2–1. Speech and Language Evaluation/Plan of Treatment

Name:		Birth Date:	
Parents:		Age:	
Address:		Evaluation Date:	
		Diagnosis:	
Phone:		Procedure:	

Background

Includes information regarding:

- maternal health
- gestational age
- birth history
- developmental milestones
- accidents, injuries, illnesses
- current medications
- previous therapy

Assessment

Results of the following tests will be given in standard scores, percentile rank, and/or age equivalency. Standard scores are a statistical score with a national average of 100 and an average performance range of 85 to 115. Scaled scores are a statistical score with a national average of 10 and an average range of 8 to 12. Percentile rank is interpreted as performance of a student that is equal to or higher than the indicated percentage of students of his or her age in a normative sample. An average percentile rank is 50 with an average range of 25 to 75. Age equivalency means that performance is comparable to the score earned by average students who were of that chronological age.

Articulation:
- List name of test administered
  - A description of what the test measures

For example:
The Structured Photographic Articulation Test II (SPAT D II) (Dawson & Tattersall, 2001) is designed to assess articulation skills in words where the sound is used by itself (e.g., carrot—

the *t* is not used with another consonant with it) and in consonant blends (sl, st, sn, etc.) and to look at the process of sound production for the rules of sounds (e.g., consonant sounds are made at the beginning of words) (Dawson & Tattersall, 2001).

- Scores obtained:

Raw Score	Standard Score	Percentile Rank	Scaled Score	Stanine	Age Equivalency

Description of the student's performance (This may include a chart showing the sounds presented and the student's error pattern.):

Receptive Vocabulary Measure:

- List name of test administered
  - A description of what the test measures

For example:
The Receptive One Word Picture Vocabulary Test (ROWPVT) (Brownell, 2011) is a test of an individual's ability to understand the meaning of single words. The individual's performance, when compared to the normative group, gives an indication of the extent of the person's English-speaking vocabulary. The test presents four color pictures per page. The examiner says a word and the student has to point to one picture from the four that represents that word (Brownell, 2011).

- Scores obtained:

Raw Score	Standard Score	Percentile Rank	Scaled Score	Stanine	Age Equivalency

Results indicate receptive vocabulary skills.

Expressive Vocabulary Measure:

- List name of test administered
  - A description of what the test measures
- Scores obtained:

Raw Score	Standard Score	Percentile Rank	Scaled Score	Stanine	Age Equivalency

continues

continued

Description of the student's performance:

For example:
Results indicate expressive vocabulary skills in the . . .

A comparison between the receptive and expressive vocabulary standard scores:
The following comparison was obtained in comparing the receptive vocabulary with the score achieved when deducting for word-finding difficulties:

Receptive Standard Score	
Expressive Standard Score	
Difference	
Statistical Significance at (whatever level)	
Significant	

A description of the significance of the scores:

For example:
According to the test manual, "lower performance on the EOWPVT as compared to the ROWPVT could mean that the individual has word-retrieval difficulties that affect the extent of his or her speaking vocabulary relative to the extent of the individual's hearing vocabulary."

Owing to the responses obtained on the expressive vocabulary test and the significant difference between the receptive and expressive vocabulary tests, a more thorough assessment of word retrieval was deemed necessary.

Test of Word Finding 2 (TWF 2)
TWF-2 provides naming tasks that were extensively researched to provide a deep assessment into the word-retrieval abilities of children (German, 2000).

Section	Raw Score	Comprehension Score
Picture Naming: Nouns		
Sentence Completion Naming		
Picture Naming: Verbs		
Picture Naming: Categories		
Total Scores		
Word-Finding Quotient		
Percentile Rank		

Description of test results:

The profile of the quotient score places this student in the below average range for her word-retrieval skills. Errors included:

- Semantically related substitution: words that are related to or co-occur with the target word such as telescope for microscope, wax for polish, pouring for watering, punching for fighting, cutting for peeling, pouring for oiling, dice for dominoes, music for instruments, carousel for Ferris wheel, chairs for furniture

- Errors based on the visual picture: chopsticks for wishbone

Word finding refers to the ability to quickly and easily retrieve a particular word from memory. Having a word-finding problem is the inability to quickly recall a word from memory even though the word is well known to the student.

Characteristics of word-finding difficulties are demonstrated by the student who may:

- use long pauses within sentences as he or she "searches" for a word

- use many vague words such as "thing" and "stuff"

- use many interjections such as "um"

- use the hands to draw in the air or act out what he or she is trying to say

- describe the word or use a similar word in the place of the word needed

- answer "I don't know" or fail to even respond to questions when it is clear that he or she does know

- have difficulty retrieving words in the presence of good comprehension of the words that he or she is unable to find (the student appears not to know answers when in reality he or she knows but is unable to express that knowledge)

- exhibit problems retrieving specific words in single-word retrieval contexts and in discourse

This student's response pattern profile is that of a slow/accurate retriever. A student who is a slow/accurate retriever is described as one who may be slower to respond in class but will provide the correct answer when he or she responds. The student may provide a similar word or response then self-correct. However, when given a choice of answers, this student is able to select the correct answer.

Language assessment:

- List name of test administered
  - A description of what the test measures
- Scores obtained:

Raw Score	Standard Score	Percentile Rank	Scaled Score	Stanine	Age Equivalency

continues

continued

A description of the student's performance, including a detailed analysis of error patterns:

For example:

If the OWLS (Carrow-Woolfolk, 1996) was presented, a detailed description of the results could include information regarding whether the student could understand receptively and expressively and produce multiple meanings of words, inferences, and figurative language.

Information Regarding Rating Scales

The Observational Rating Scale (ORS) is a scale completed by a parent, teacher, or student to identify contexts or situations in which the student demonstrates difficulty with language (Semel, Wiig, & Secord, 1995). This scale was completed by _____.

The following areas were scored as occurring often or always:

    Speaking:

    Listening:

    Reading:

    Writing:

Language Processing Testing

- List name of test administered
  - A description of what the test measures
- Scores obtained:

Subtest Name	Raw Score	Scaled Score	Percentile Rank

	Overall	Phonologic	Memory	Cohesion
Sum of Scaled Scores				
Index Standard Scores				

Other tests administered:

Summary:

Plan of Treatment:

Recommendations:

Long-Term Goals:

Short-Term Goals:

Prognosis:

Frequency/Duration:

Home Ideas:

1. Make a card file to keep new vocabulary words so that they can be rehearsed daily.
2. Obtain pleasure books or books assigned for school on tape so that the student can listen and read at the same time to increase overall comprehension.

Accommodation suggestions for school:

1. Preferential seating with no visual or auditory distractions, including fluorescent light noise, heater noise, appropriate lighting, appropriate temperature, etc.
2. Chunk information and directions. Provide directions in a simplified form.
3. Provide key words and a subject outline on the board for directions.
4. Provide structured strategies for word finding to assist in retrieval of information (refer to #1 category, function, location/origin).
5. Call on the student as soon as the student's hand goes up so he or she does not lose the thought.
6. Highlight or use symbols with color coding to reinforce directions.
7. Wait for the count of 10 one thousands when asking a question so that the student has time to process it; reinforce the student positively when difficulty arises.
8. Provide extended time for tests and the availability for a professional to assist with understanding of directions and to assess for understanding.
9. Provide a word bank for open-ended test questions.
10. Allow the student to turn in written assignments to the teacher or resource for review and discussion before turning in for a final grade (may turn in for a grade but then is given the opportunity to correct errors; this would then be graded again and the two grades would be combined for a final grade).
11. Allow the student to read along if the teacher is reading from a book or text.
12. Assign a buddy note taker so that the student can have a copy of this student's note if needed (e.g., lecture, absence, etc.)

Signature

Title

Conclusion

The diagnostic process is more than determining what tests to administer. It begins with assessing what difficulties the student is having academically. By assessing the profile, the speech-language pathologist can determine what tests should be administered. The evaluation should include at least a measure of receptive and expressive vocabulary and language skills and an assessment of word finding. Further tests or assessments by other professionals, such as an audiologist, may be necessary based on the information obtained during these tests. The second step is to determine where the deficits are. This should be based on clinical observation, expertise, and judgment during the testing as well as assessing each individual subtest of any battery. Once the profile is complete, the evaluation report should include a description of the student's background, information regarding understanding standard scores, a list and description of the tests used, and specific results and clinical observations during each specific test administered. This information should be summarized followed by impressions, recommendations, and goals.

A complete diagnostic assessment is critical to determining areas for remediation. We can hold the key to academic success for a student. The first step is a comprehensive evaluation.

References

Bellis, T., Chermak, G., Ferre, J., Musiek, F., Rosenberg, G., & Williams, E. (2005). *(Central) auditory processing disorders*. Rockville, MD: American Speech-Language-Hearing Association.

Bowers, L., Huisingh, R., & LoGiudice, C. (2004). *Test of Problem Solving 2—Adolescent*. East Moline, IL: LinguiSystems.

Bowers, L., Huisingh, R., & LoGiudice, C. (2005). *Test of Problem Solving 3—Elementary (TOPS)*. East Moline, IL: LinguiSystems.

Brownell, R. (2011). *Expressive One Word Picture Vocabulary Test* (4 ed.). Novato, CA: Academic Therapy Publications.

Brownell, R. (2011). *Receptive One Word Picture Vocabulary Test* (4 ed.). Novato, CA: Academic Therapy Publications.

Carrow-Woolfolk, E. (1996). *Oral Written Language Scales (OWLS)*. Bloomington, MN: AGS.

Carrow-Woolfolk, E. (1999). *Comprehensive Assessment of Spoken Language*. San Antonio, TX: Pearson.

Dawson, J., & Tattersall, P. (2001). *Structured Photo Articulation Test II*. DeKalb, IL: Janelle Publications.

Dunn, D. M., & Dunn, L. M. (2007). *Peabody Picture Vocabulary Test, Fourth Edition (PPVT4)* San Antonio, TX: Pearson Assessments.

Fisher, L. I. (1985). Learning disabilities and auditory processing. In R. J. Van Hattum (Ed.), *Administration of speech-language services in the schools* (pp. 231–292). San Diego, CA: College Hill Press.

German, D. (1990). *Test of Adolescent/Adult Word Finding (TAWF)*. Austin, TX: Pro-Ed.

German, D. (1991). *Test of Word Finding in Discourse*. Austin, TX: Pro-Ed.

German, D. (2000). *Test of Word Finding II (TWF II)*. Austin, TX: Pro-Ed.

German, D. (2009, November 20). *Tier 2 dual focus vocabulary instruction for learners with word finding disabilities*. Lecture conducted at the American Speech-Language-Hearing Association National Convention, New Orleans, LA.

Gillon, G. (2002, December 3). Phonological awareness intervention for children: From the research laboratory to the clinic. *The ASHA Leader,* 1.

Hadley, P. (1998). Language sampling protocols for eliciting text-level discourse. *Language,*

Speech, and Hearing Services in Schools, 29, 132–147.

Hammill, D., Brown, V., & Larsen, S. (2009). *Test of Written Language 4*. Austin, TX: Pro-Ed.

Hammill, D., Brown, V., Larsen, S., & Wiederholt, J. L. (2007). *Test of Adolescent and Adult Language* (4th ed.). Austin, TX: Pro-Ed.

Hammill, D., & Newcomer, P. (2008). *Test of Language Development—Intermediate* (4th ed.). Austin, TX: Pro-Ed.

Herron, S., Hresko, W., & Peak, P. (2001). *Test of Early Written Language TEWL-2 (Complete kit)* (null ed.). Austin, TX: Pro-Ed.

Invernizzi, M. (2004). *Phonological Awareness and Literacy Screening (PALS)*. Charlottesville: The Rector and The Board of Visitors of the University of Virginia.

Keith, R. (2009). *SCAN 3A*. San Antonio, TX: Pearson.

Keith, R. (2009). *SCAN 3C*. San Antonio, TX: Pearson.

Martin, N., & Brownell, R. (2005). *Test of Auditory Processing Skills 3 (TAPS 3)*. Novato, CA: Academic Therapy Publications.

Nickisch, A., & Kries, R. V. (2009). Short-term memory (STM) constraints in children with specific language impairment (SLI): Are there differences between receptive and expressive SLI? *Journal of Speech, Language, and Hearing Research, 52,* 578–595.

Nunes, T., Bryant, P., & Bindman, M. (2006). The effects of learning to spell on children's awareness of morphology. *Reading and Writing: An Interdisciplinary Journal, 19*(7), 767–787.

Richard, G., & Ferre, J. (2006). *Differential Screening Test for Processing*. East Moline, IL: LinguiSystems.

Robertson, C., & Salter, W. (1995). *Phonological Awareness Profile*. East Moline, IL: LinguiSystems.

Robertson, C., & Salter, W. (2007). *Phonological Awareness Test 2*. East Moline, IL: LinguiSystems.

Schmidek, D. H. (1997). *Guide to narrative language: Procedures for assessment*. Greenville, SC: Super Duper Publications.

Semel, E., Wiig, E., & Secord, W. (1995). *Clinical Evaluation of Language Fundamentals 3 (CELF-3) Observational Rating Scale*. San Antonio, TX: Pearson.

Semel, E., Wiig, E., & Secord, W. (2003). *Clinical Evaluation of Language Fundamentals 4*. San Antonio, TX: Pearson.

Semel, E., Wiig, E., & Secord, W. (2004). *Clinical Evaluation of Language Fundamentals—Preschool* (2nd ed.). San Antonio, TX: Pearson.

Shipley, K., Stone, T., & Sue, B. (1983). *Test for Examining Expressive Morphology*. Austin, TX: Pro-Ed.

Sittner Bridges, M., & Catts, H. (2011). *Dynamic Screening for Phonological Awareness*. East Moline, IL: LinguiSystems.

Torgesen, J., Wagner, R., & Rashotte, C. (1997). Prevention and remediation of severe reading disabilities: Keeping the end in mind. *Scientific Studies of Reading, 1,* 217–234.

Torgesen, J. K., & Bryant, B. R. (2004). *Test of Phonological Awareness TOPA 2+ Plus (Complete kit)*. Austin, TX: Pro-Ed.

Wagner, R., Torgesen, J., & Rashotte, C. (1999). *Comprehensive Test of Phonological Processing CTOPP (Complete kit)*. Austin, TX: Pro-Ed.

Wallace, G., & Hammill, D. (2008). *Crevt-2: Comprehensive Receptive and Expressive Vocabulary Test—Second Edition*. Austin, TX: Pro-Ed.

Wechsler, D. (2009). *Wechsler Individual Achievement Test III* (3rd ed.). Austin, TX: Pro-Ed.

Williams, K. (2007). *Expressive Vocabulary Test Second Edition*. San Antonio, TX: Riverside.

Wolf Nelson, N., Catts, H., Ehren, B., Roth, F., Scott, C., & Staskowski, M. (2001). *Roles and responsibilities of speech-language pathologist with respect to reading and writing in children* [Position statement]. Rockville, MD: American Speech-Language-Hearing Association.

Woodcock, R., McGrew, K., & Mather, N. (2001). *Woodcock-Johnson III—Tests of Achievement* (3rd ed.). Rolling Meadows, IL: Riverside.

Zimmerman, I. L., Steiner, V. G., & Pond, R. E. (2002). *Preschool Language Scale 4 (PLS 4)*. San Antonio, TX: Pearson.

Zimmerman, I. L., Steiner, V. G., & Pond, R. E. (2005). *Preschool Language Scale 4 Screening Test (PLS 4 Screening Test)*. San Antonio, TX: Pearson.

Zimmerman, I. L., Steiner, V. G., & Pond, R. E. (2011). *Preschool Language Scale 5 (PLS 5)*. San Antonio, TX: Pearson.

3

Getting Started: Preliteracy Skills

Introduction

As stated in chapter 1, many children with reading problems have spoken language problems (Reed, 2005). Language impairment and reading disorders commonly co-occur with an auditory processing disorder (APD) (Sharma, Purdy, & Kelly, 2009). It is important to understand language milestones in preschool and kindergarten and the impact that nonmastery of these milestones may have on learning and literacy skills. These milestones should have special consideration as we set our goals. When evaluating the language skills of a preschooler or kindergarten student, we must look for milestones that are not mastered and that may be indicators of emerging literacy or other skills needed for later academic success. Even though a child's overall score may be within a higher age level or even within the expected range for the child's chronological age, milestones that are not mastered may be an issue. Certain missing skills may be skills that are very important for emerging literacy skills (prealphabetic and early phonetic) and overall academic success.

In the American Speech-Language-Hearing Association (ASHA) Guidelines for Early Intervention, several areas of the document (Function of the SLP, Word Production and Word Combinations, and Emergent Literacy) state how speech and/or language delay has an impact on emerging literacy and future academic success. ASHA's Guidelines for Early Intervention include vocabulary under Word Production and Word Combinations. Preschooler or kindergarten students with delays in receptive vocabulary development may demonstrate difficulty understanding age-appropriate words when the words are heard in stories, in the context of directions, and later in classroom activities (Wilcox et al., 2008).

Another area that should be monitored with preschool- and kindergarten-age children is their ability to follow directions of increasing length and complexity. The ability to follow directions moves from being able to follow one-step familiar directions to one-step unfamiliar directions. Two-step directions move from two-step related directions where the preschooler or kindergarten student could follow the direction, even if part of the direction was omitted, to following two-step unrelated directions. Following directions relies on auditory short-term memory. Auditory short-term memory is needed to understand directions at home and later in the classroom setting. It also is needed to hold information into term memory long enough to manipulate the information for comprehension and reasoning. Therefore, difficulty following directions or repeating information verbatim in the preschool years or in kindergarten could indicate difficulty with auditory short-term memory skills that will have an academic impact.

> **Auditory short-term memory:** The ability to hold auditory information into memory for a short duration of time.

Lastly, narrative development has been found to impact literacy development and academic achievement significantly (Dickinson & Tabors, 2001). Retelling of a story requires language comprehension, memory, and strong oral language skills (Hughes, McGillivray, & Schmidek, 1997). Research further shows that children who enter kindergarten with sophisticated narrative skills have an educational advantage (Snow, Tabors, Nicholson, & Kurland, 1995).

For preschool children and kindergarten students who are demonstrating expressive language delay, a delay in producing sounds, developing vocabulary skills, asking and answering questions, understanding and using grammatical markers, understanding verb tenses, developing quantity concepts, and retelling events also could have an impact on later academic success. For example, difficulty retelling events may be an indication of difficulty with sequencing or understanding the concepts that signify a sequence of events (before, during, after, first, second, last). A child needs to be able to sequence events in order to understand the order that a direction should be followed, to understand the order of activities for the day, and later to retell a story in the order that he or she has read. A significant decrease in expressive vocabulary scores on a vocabulary test as compared to higher receptive vocabulary scores also is an indicator of possible word-finding difficulties.

Word finding can have a significant impact on a child's academic progress. According to McGregor (1997), preschool children with a word-finding disorder produce more errors in single word naming and in discourse. Errors are typically semantic or perceptual (visual) versus phonological. Preschool or kindergarten children with word-finding difficulties often demonstrate difficulty with expressing (recalling) beginning concepts, such as color words and shapes, when mastery of these skills is expected. Retrieval difficulties on rapid automatic naming of category vocabulary (household items, toys, animals) can be observed in these children as well. The next skill set that typically is affected by word finding is the ability to recall alphabet letters, sounds of the letters, and sight words. This is demonstrated in written expression when these children enter school as they need to recall the alphabet letters in words or a known word as a whole.

It is important for us to attempt to identify why the preschooler or kindergarten student is experiencing language or speech delays. For example, if a preschooler or kindergarten student is demonstrating difficulty following auditory directions or repeating words and sentences verbatim, the student may be demonstrating difficulty with auditory short-term memory, which would lead to difficulty following auditory directions in a classroom, remembering details of a story read in class, following classroom discussions, and learning new skills that are verbally taught by the teacher.

If a preschooler or kindergarten student is demonstrating a significant gap between receptive and expressive language, atypical sound errors, consonant voicing errors, and vowel errors, Childhood Apraxia of Speech (CAS) should be considered. The Childhood Apraxia of Speech Association of North America (CASANA) states that children with a diagnosis of CAS are at high risk for literacy problems and language-learning related educational difficulties (CASANA, n.d.). Preschool children with CAS and a comorbid language disorder often demonstrate difficulty with expressive language. This includes difficulties with morphology and phonology, which are skills needed for future academic success. Parents frequently report that their preschooler or kindergarten student said a word once or twice then did not say it again. This also is another early indicator of CAS difficulties. It is my experience that these are the students who should be monitored closely for word-finding difficulties later.

It is vital for a speech-language pathologist who works only with preschool children (birth to 3 years of age) to be able to advise parents regarding what to look for as their preschooler moves toward prekindergarten and kindergarten age. Early language mastery and demonstration of preliteracy skills such as phonological awareness skills are all indicators of later reading and academic success.

Phonological awareness: Understanding of word sound structure and how it can be broken down into smaller units. It includes segmenting words into syllables, segmenting words into individual sounds, identifying individual sounds in words, identifying and producing rhyming words, and blending sounds to make words.

A vast number of the strategies discussed in this chapter are appropriate through kindergarten, and possibly beyond, based on the skill level of the child. Response to Intervention calls for educators to differentiate instruction based on students' skill level. Many of the strategies are appropriate for all tiers of intervention. There are great strategies that can be incorporated into a daily kindergarten program (Tier I), some that would work well in a small group (Tier II), and others that are excellent for Tier III intensive individual intervention. Many of the strategies include other modalities of input such as tactile, visual, or kinesthetic.

This chapter also addresses goals and strategies that can be used with preschool through kindergarten children to encourage skills needed for reading and academic success. The strategies presented in this chapter assist with the areas of auditory short-term memory, sequencing, word finding, phonological awareness, and narrative skills for the preschool child.

Auditory Short-Term Memory Introduction

As discussed previously, the speech-language pathologist assesses areas that may indicate difficulties with auditory short-term memory even when working with very young preschool children. Zimmerman, Steiner, and Pond (2002) and Rossetti (1990) provide the following developmental milestones that relate to auditory short-term memory. These are listed within the 3-month intervals of test items:

- 9–12 months: Follows simple commands occasionally
- 12–15 months: Follows one-step directions during play
- 21–24 months: Follows novel commands and follows two-step related commands
- 30–33 months: Follows two-step unrelated commands
- 33–36 months: Follows a three-step unrelated command; listens attentively to a short story
- 36–42 months: Follows directions with two objects or two actions
- 42–48 months: Can retell a story after listening to it
- 53–59 months: Repeats sentences verbatim

These milestones need to be monitored for acquisition, especially if they are the only milestones within a developmental age range that have not been mastered. In my experience, this may indicate that auditory short-term memory skills may not be developing along with the other skills. For a young child, age-appropriate auditory short-term memory skills are necessary for following directions, remembering a story that is read, and remembering songs and finger plays. Age-appropriate auditory short-term memory skills also are needed for following the directions of a classroom teacher; remembering the activities of the day; and as the child progresses in grade level, remembering classroom lecture information and homework assignments.

Area: Auditory Short-Term Memory

Examples of Goals

The preschooler or kindergarten student will:

1. increase the ability to hold a series of related words in short-term memory
2. increase the ability to repeat sentences verbatim with and without a visual cue
3. follow directions of increasing length and complexity
4. retell a favorite story with and without visual cues

5. retell a story heard for the first time

6. follow auditory directions with increasing length and complexity

Rationale: It is necessary for preschool or kindergarten students to develop auditory short-term memory skills in order to have academic success later. These students must be able to follow classroom instructions and gain new knowledge from the teacher. It also is important to be able to hold auditory information in short-term memory in order to manipulate the information for auditory comprehension. This will assist with following written directions and reading comprehension, which rely on visual short-term memory in the future.

Auditory Short-Term Memory Strategies

Strategy 1: Here's How to Use Books

Step 1: Use books with flaps or textures.

In my experience I typically can get a preschooler or kindergarten student to look at books if the pictures are not overly stimulating and if he or she can manipulate the book. I find that flap books usually work better than textured books initially. Once I get the preschooler or kindergarten student's attention to flap books, textured books work the best as the next step. Again, textured books with minimal words and visual stimulation should be targeted first. These books typically have one to two sentences per page. The child then has to look under the flap to find the item discussed. The ability to listen to the simple sentences will assist with auditory short-term memory.

Step 2: Use books with repeating phrases.

Books that provide a repetitive phrase will hold the attention of the preschooler and kindergarten student as well as increase auditory short-term memory for the repeated information.

Step 3: Use books with onset and rime words.

> **Onset and rime:** In a syllable, the onset is the initial consonant or consonants, and the rime is the vowel and any consonants that follow it (e.g., in the word *cat*, the onset is "c" and the rime is "at").

By providing books with rhyming words, it is hoped that the preschooler or kindergarten student will be more involved due to the change in adult intonation, which is needed while reading these types of books. It also will familiarize them with the pattern of onset and rime words (a phonological awareness skill) as a needed preliteracy skill.

Step 4: Use stand-alone pictures with books.

Any objects or pictures that the preschooler or kindergarten student can manipulate while listening will increase his or her attention to the book—thus, to the auditory information. This includes books such as Mayer-Johnson adaptive books, educator-made materials, to felt story books.

Strategy 2: Here's How to Use Visual Strategies for Preparation of Auditory Input

As preschoolers get closer to kindergarten, they will need to be able to attend to more auditory information at one time due to the setup of a classroom environment. Enhancement of visual strategies can assist with organization of a room, an event, a center in the classroom, or a worksheet. If a child is visually attentive, it is hoped that when auditory information is presented, the child does not need to scan the page, center, or room while listening to auditory information. If the preschooler or kindergarten student can visualize first, then he or she is ready to listen to auditory information without needing to attempt to visualize and listen at the same time.

Step 1: Find pictures that can be divided easily.

Find pictures that can be divided easily into four equal sections (quadrants). *Processing Auditory Information Exactly and Totally* (DeGaetano, 1994) provides pictures that are easily divided to use this strategy.

Step 2: Get the main idea.

Assist the preschooler or kindergarten student in looking at the picture as a whole while visually scanning from left to right (a skill later needed for reading and writing) and attempting to decide what the main idea of the picture is. The speech-language pathologist can ask, "If you were to give the picture a title, what would it be?"

Step 3: Divide the picture into quadrants and in half.

1. First, the speech-language pathologist demonstrates how to divide the picture into quadrants in order to view the sections. This may take a couple of sessions.

2. Then the speech-language pathologist asks the preschooler or kindergarten student to use a finger to show where the lines should go and then divides the sheet by folding or using a pencil to draw lines to divide.

3. Upon success with step 2, the student divides the sheet into the four sections by folding or using a crayon or pencil to divide the picture.

4. After splitting the picture into quadrants successfully and providing great detail about each quadrant as described in step 5, the student divides the sheet in half to assist with visually scanning a greater area of the picture.

5. The student visually scans the sheet from left to right as if the lines were present.

Step 4: Discuss the page by quadrant, half, and whole.

1. The speech-language pathologist leads the preschooler or kindergarten student to discuss the upper left, the upper right, the bottom left, and finally the bottom right. He or she then asks questions for the child to describe the picture. For example, the speech-language pathologist might say, "What animals do you see in this section?" "What are the cows doing?"

2. When the student has progressed to splitting the paper in half, the speech-language pathologist discusses the top half, progressing from left to right, then the bottom half.

3. The preschooler or kindergarten student then visualizes the entire paper by scanning left to right to discuss the page in its entirety.

Step 5: Gain knowledge about the picture. The speech-language pathologist assists the preschooler or kindergarten student by:

1. turning over the paper and asking the student to describe each quadrant of the paper

2. asking questions to assist the student with obtaining the main idea of the picture, which relates back to the title given to the page. This can be accomplished by asking the student, "If you were going to make up a story about this picture, what would you call the story?"

3. asking questions to assist the student with obtaining at least three details to support the main idea

Step 6: Follow auditory directions. The speech-language pathologist assists the preschooler or kindergarten student:

1. by making sure that materials needed to complete directions are organized before presenting the directions

2. by presenting his or her directions or those provided with the picture. The directions increase in length and complexity as the preschooler or kindergarten student successfully follows less difficult directions.

3. with reorganizing materials after each direction is followed. This way the student is not searching for the right color crayon when he or she should be focused on the auditory information.

The goal is for the preschooler or kindergarten student to be able to move left to right through the page (necessary for reading and writing) and divide a room, worksheet, or any visual scene in sections to understand the visual information better. This also is useful for an area that is visually overstimulating or difficult to organize for a preschooler and kindergarten student. If a preschooler or kindergarten student needs to clean up a room, the room can be divided into quadrants in order to visualize just a section so that the student will be able to move productively through the room. The picture or area can be divided just as easily into two sections by visualizing the dividing line through the middle top to bottom versus side to side.

Strategy 3: Here's How to Use Visualizing to Assist With Recall

The goal is to help the preschooler or kindergarten student visualize a place in order to categorize items and assist with recall of a group of words.

Step 1: Pick a place that the preschooler or kindergarten student knows well.
This could be the student's house, a particular room, or a frequently visited place (zoo, store, library).

Step 2: Have the preschooler or kindergarten student enter the door and tell what is seen.
In this step, the preschooler or kindergarten student can randomly tell what is seen.

Step 3: Assist the preschooler or kindergarten student with organizing the space.
The adult assists the preschooler or kindergarten student in dividing the room into quadrants or halves depending on the space and how much visual information the student can absorb at any one time.

The adult should assist the child scan 360 degrees, like moving around a clock, beginning from where the child is standing.

Step 4: Recall items.
Once the preschooler or kindergarten student can build a visually organized picture to describe the space, the adult can provide a series of items for the preschooler or kindergarten student to recall in the order that they are found in the space.

1. A room in the house: "Walk through the living room and pretend you are getting a pillow off the couch, a book from the book rack, candle from the sofa table, and the remote from the television." "Tell me the four items you are getting in the order that you would find them in the room."

2. Enter into a store: "You need to get toothpaste, shampoo, gardening gloves, a paint brush, a toy car, and a gallon of milk."

Besides working to increase auditory short-term memory through visual strategies, a second benefit to the preceding strategies is that they also will begin to teach the preschooler and kindergarten student organizational skills. The student learns how to visually organize worksheets, books, or other materials that will be used in a classroom by knowing how to visually divide the sheet into sections. The student can better put toys away in the playroom if he or she can visually look at the room in sections and begin organizing that section. It is important to teach preschooler and kindergarten students beginning organizational skills so that they are not searching for toys, crayons, scissors, or other such objects and are ready to be active listeners. Other activities to assist in this organization include using transparent storage containers with lids to organize the preschooler and kindergarten students' room and play area. The containers can have a picture of the toy on it so that they know what is in the bin. Preschooler or kindergarten students can be encouraged to play with one bin and clean up before getting out another bin. At school, a pencil box with only the items needed can be used. These students should be encouraged to place the items back in the box so the utensil can be found easily when listening to the next direction.

Strategy 4: Here's How to Retell Familiar Stories by Looking at the Pictures

Step 1: Retell a previously read story to the preschooler and kindergarten student.
The adult chooses one of the preschooler and kindergarten student's favorite books to read.

Step 2: Look at the pictures and retell the story.
The adult turns the pages as the preschooler or kindergarten student retells the story by looking at the pictures. The adult may have to assist the student in figuring out the main idea of the story and the details that support the main idea.

Strategy 5: Here's How to Retell Unfamiliar Stories by Looking at the Pictures

Step 1: Read a story that is unfamiliar to the preschooler or kindergarten student.
The adult chooses a story to read that the student has not heard.

Step 2: Have the preschooler or kindergarten student look at the pictures and retell the story.
After the adult reads the story, the student is assisted with turning the pages while looking at the pictures and tells what he or she can remember from the story. The adult may have to use questions to assist the child with recalling the information. Owing to the student's auditory short-term memory limitations, the adult also may have to read a section of the book and review that section with the student before the next section is read. Again, the preschooler or kindergarten student may need assistance in figuring out the main idea of the story and in providing supporting details.

Strategy 6: Here's How to Use Songs and Finger Plays to Increase Auditory Short-Term Memory

The speech-language pathologist or educator is encouraged to use either already made materials to visually support songs and finger plays or make materials to support the songs and finger plays. I typically use a permanent marker or label maker to add the name of the picture on the object in order to familiarize the preschooler or kindergarten student with the printed word representing the object.

Step 1: Use an already made book that includes a variety of preschool stories and songs. These types of books have objects that preschooler or kindergarten students can manipulate while participating in the story. There are classics such as *Gingerbread Man, Three Little Pigs,* and *Five Little Monkeys.* There also are category books based around weather, town, school, bedtime, and shopping. Song books include "Old MacDonald" and "Wheels on the Bus."

Step 2: Make key pictures to support the auditory short-term memory. The child can manipulate pictures while participating in the story. Pictures can be acquired through products such as Mayer-Johnson's Board Maker (n.d.), Therasimplicity's Sound Mapping (n.d.), Do to Learn's Make a Schedule (n.d.), Google images, or other icon makers. With the author's or publisher's permission, pictures from the actual book can be photocopied and laminated to use during the story.

Foam board also can be used to create manipulatives. For example, for the song "I Know a Lady Who Swallowed a Fly," a picture of a woman can be drawn on the foam board with the middle cut out to attach a cloth bag. Toys (a spider, a fly, a bird, a cat, a dog, a cow, and a horse) could then be put in the cloth bag as the song is sung. I always change the words to "I bet she'll cry."

Step 3: Use popular songs and finger plays as manipulatives. Words are available on various Web sites such as KIDiddles (n.d.). Search lyrics to these children's songs:

- "Wheels on the Bus"
- "Old MacDonald"
- Old MacDonald for vowels. A great way to help preschool and kindergarten children to distinguish vowels from consonants is to use the tune of "Old MacDonald," but instead of animals vowels are used: "Old MacDonald had a vowel, /a/, /e/, /i/, /o/, /u/ and sometimes /y/."
- "There's a Hole in My Bucket"
- "Five Little Ducks"
- "Hokey Pokey"

These can then be used as manipulatives to assist preschooler or kindergarten students with retelling or resinging the songs and finger plays. Velcro strips on a white board make a great working surface for the students to be able to re-create the story or song sequence.

Strategy 7: Here's How to Use Games to Increase Auditory Short-Term Memory

A variety of games can be used to increase auditory short-term memory:

1. Telephone Game: The preschooler or kindergarten student whispers a given message in the next student's ear, and that student has to relay the exact message to the next student. The last student says the message that he or she heard aloud.

2. Alphabet Game for Kindergartners: The game starts with the first letter of the alphabet with the first player stating, "My name is _____, and my brother's name is _____. We live in _____ and we sell _____."

   For example: My name is Alicia, and my brother's name is Alex. We live in Arkansas and we sell antiques. The next player repeats what the previous player had said and goes through the sentences with B words and so on. Each player must repeat all of the information provided by all previous players before adding the next letter's information.

Other examples are:

- "I went to the _____ (store, beach, moon, camp, zoo, farm, etc.), and I took . . . " Each player repeats the previously stated items and adds another item.

- Simon Says. Each player takes a turn being the one giving the directions, or the adult can give the directions. The preschooler or kindergarten student has to wait for "Simon Says" then follow the direction. If the direction does not include "Simon Says" then the student does not follow the direction. The directions can increase in complexity.

In conclusion, increasing auditory short-term memory skills through visual strategies assists preschooler or kindergarten students with using the environment in order to gain greater visual information to support what is being provided auditorally.

Sequencing Events Introduction

By 36 months, preschooler students should be able to relate past experiences verbally (Rossetti, 1990). This includes being able to tell at least a couple of activities that occurred in a day. The ability to sequence past events means that the preschooler or kindergarten students are beginning to understand activities that occurred in the past. Being able to sequence past activities will lead to these students being able to retell a story. Next, they will be able to relate activities that will happen. This will lead to understanding activities that will occur in the future as well as begin making inferences and predictions regarding what will happen. Preschooler or kindergarten students must understand sequencing of events before being expected to understand left-to-right progression for reading words in a sentence or sounding out the sequence of sounds in a word.

Area: Sequencing of Events

Examples of Goals

The preschooler or kindergarten student will:

1. understand and use past and future tense verbs expressively in order to comprehend past events and events that will occur in the future

2. understand time/sequence vocabulary, including times of the day, seasons of the year, and order (first, second, third, beginning, middle, end)

3. produce time/sequence vocabulary, including times of the day, seasons of the year, and order (first, second, third, beginning, middle, end)

4. sequence a past event, including increasing amounts of information in the correct order.

5. tell about an event that will occur in the order that it will occur

6. retell a story in the correct order

Rationale: By 36 months, preschoolers should be able to relate past events. According to the Preschool Language Scale-4 (PLS-4), a child whose skill is listed at the 6:6 to 6:11 skill area should be able to tell a story with an introduction, sequence of steps, and a conclusion. This may start as simply telling one or two events that occurred when a parent was not present. Preschooler or kindergarten students need to understand time concepts, including times of the day or seasons of the year (4½-year-old skill area on the PLS-4). These students also must understand the time/sequence concepts of first, second, third (5½-year-old skill area on the PLS-4). Preschooler or kindergarten students need to understand the following: sequencing, in order to follow directions in the correct order; the order that events will occur throughout the day; the calendar; and, most importantly, that sounds in a certain sequential pattern make up a word.

Sequencing Strategies

Strategy 1: Here's How to Use Schedule Boards to Retell a Day's Events

A schedule board can be made and used in preschool and beyond to recall and sequence events of the day. It can be set up so that it can be printed and the teacher can write in a few key words for each event (Table 3–1).

1. Use pictures to represent the events of the day.
2. Leave room for the teacher or parent to write one or two events that occurred during that time.
3. The speech-language pathologist, parent, or other adult working with the preschooler or kindergarten student can then show the pictures for the student to recall what happened during that time.

Table 3–1. Event Board

My Day	
Preschooler's Name: Date:	
👪 Group Meeting	Calendar: Weather:
📖 Story Time	Story name: The story was about:
✂️ ✏️ Craft Time	We made . . .
🍽️ Snack Time	Food: Drink:
📄 Writing/Journal	

This will decrease the amount of writing that the teacher has to complete for each preschooler and kindergarten student. It provides the speech-language pathologist, parent, or other adult working with the preschooler or kindergarten student a means to ask questions about the student's day if the student is unable to recall events and/or provide the correct sequence for the day.

Strategy 2: Here's How to Sequence Story Cards

1. Already made sequencing cards can be used to assist preschooler or kindergarten students in understanding the order in which an event can occur. These cards are usually available in 3- to 6-step sequences and are available from education stores. If a preschooler or kindergarten student is having difficulty with sequencing, it may be advantageous to present the final picture

so that he or she can understand the big picture. Then the student can place the remaining pictures in the correct order from the beginning of the story.

2. Pictures can also be cut from magazines or obtained online to provide sequences for stories.

Strategy 3: Here's How to Sequence Daily Activities

For daily events such as getting ready for school and for routines such as lunch or dinner time and bedtime, special activities can be drawn or pictures used in order to assist the preschooler or kindergarten student with the correct sequence of events for the activities. The student can then use this board to sequence the activity orally.

Strategy 4: Here's How to Sequence the Steps for Playing a Game

Board games to activities in gym class have a sequence of how the game is played. Visual supports also can be added to assist with retelling the sequence of steps.

Step 1: The adult explains the rules of a new game to the child.

Step 2: The child reiterates the steps in order.

Step 3: The child tell the steps for a familiar game without the adult having to explain first.

Strategy 5: Here's How to Use Crafts/Art Projects for Sequencing

Craft activities can range from very simple projects to very complex ones. A visual demonstration can be provided as the steps to complete the project are given.

Step 1: The adult explains the craft using the visual pictures.

Step 2: The child reiterates the steps in order.

Step 3: The child directs a familiar craft without the adult having to provide the steps.

Strategy 6: Here's How to Use Cooking Projects to Sequence

Using preschool children's cookbooks that provide pictures with each step is a way for the preschooler or kindergarten student to follow the recipe in the correct order. The speech-language pathologist is encouraged to either find cookbooks, such as *Kinder Krunchies* by Usborne Books, which has pictures to go with the steps in the recipes, or make icons or pictures that support the steps.

In conclusion, the ability to sequence is important for academic success. This process begins with understanding and producing past tense and future tense verbs in order to describe an event that occurred in the past or will occur in the future. The preschooler or kindergarten student is then able to relate experiences that have occurred, which leads to retelling a story and to understanding the main idea and details of that story. This is important for auditory comprehension of events in a classroom; that is, to understanding the main idea and important details of information that is read.

Phonological Awareness Introduction

Phonological awareness can be defined as the understanding of a word's sound structure. Phonological awareness can include:

- Rhyming awareness including onset and rime
- Segmenting sentences into words
- Segmenting words into syllables
- Segmenting words into individual sounds
- Identifying individual sounds in words (phonemic awareness)

> **Phonemic awareness:** The ability to hear the individual (phonemes) that make up words and the understanding that words are composed of segments of sounds smaller than syllables.

- Blending sounds to make words

Children's phonological awareness ability at preschool is a powerful predictor of later reading and writing success (Bradley & Bryant, 1983; Lundberg, Olofsson, & Wall, 1980; Torgesen, Wagner, & Rashotte, 1994).

One must have an understanding of phonological awareness in order to move toward understanding phonics. This section concentrates on the key areas in the preschool and kindergarten years that are important for phonological awareness.

> **Phonics:** Teaching how to connect the sounds of letters or groups of letters (e.g., /c/, /k/, /ck/) and how to blend the sounds of letters together to produce unknown words.

Area: Phonological Awareness

Examples of Goals

The preschooler or kindergarten student will:

1. increase understanding of onset and rime words
2. increase the ability to express onset and rime words
3. increase awareness of word families based on onset and rime

4. increase the ability to determine words in a sentence

5. increase the ability to determine syllables in words

6. increase the ability to determine sounds in a word

7. discriminate speech sounds accurately

8. discriminate words as same or different

9. produce vowel and consonant sounds accurately

Rationale: It has been said that preschool children today have difficulty with the phonological awareness of rhyming words because parents and educators no longer recite nursery rhymes or sing the rhyming songs of yesterday. There probably is a good reason for that. Today's culture is not as accepting of "a lady who lived in a shoe and had so many children she didn't know what to do" or of "little Jack Horner who sat in the corner." What about "rocka by baby in a tree top"? But the point is well taken. An opportunity to introduce rhyming words at a very early age has been decreased significantly. The implications can be huge. The ability to understand and produce rhyming words is one of the foundations of phonological awareness because of the direct impact on decoding and understanding word families.

Many preschool children, especially those with phonological awareness difficulties, demonstrate difficulty with understanding and producing rhyming words. Sometimes it will be in kindergarten or first grade before the link is made that words rhyme. I have seen children with severe CAS with a comorbid language disability who are in second grade before they understand that word families represent words that rhyme. This difficulty with rhyming words will significantly impact the child's ability to understand onset and rimes (the onset is the initial consonant or consonants, and the rime is the vowel and any consonants that follow it). These also are referred to as word families as letters are introduced (at, cat, bat, hat, rat, sat, pat, fat, mat). This will affect the preschooler or kindergarten student's proficiency in recognizing the word family in printed words. In addition it will affect this student's ability to recognize these as segments in a longer word later, thus potentially having an effect on reading accuracy and fluency.

Strategies for Phonological Awareness

Strategy 1: Here's How to Introduce Rhyming With Children

Step 1: Rhyme in everyday play.

Parents and caregivers often use rhymes and may not necessarily realize it. In doing this, parents and caregivers are beginning an important language process with their young child. Examples are:

- "Peek a Boo I See You"
- "Pat a Cake"
- "Baa Baa Black Sheep"

As the child gets older, songs that he or she will learn and be able to participate in while singing can be used.

Step 2: Use songs that rhyme for preschool children.

The perfect opportunity to introduce songs that rhyme is as a caregiver is holding and rocking a preschooler or kindergarten student. The following is a brief sample of songs and finger plays that have lasted lifetimes (and include lyrics that parents are willing to use today):

- "Hush Little Baby Don't You Cry"
- "A Tisket A Tasket"
- "Twinkle Twinkle Little Star"
- "Rain Rain Go Away"
- "Row Row Row Your Boat"
- "Do Your Ears Hang Low"
- "I Love You, You Love Me" (PBS Kids, n.d.)

Step 3: Use participation songs for preschool through first grade to assist with rhyming (Table 3–2).

- "Three Little Ducks"
  3 little ducks went out to play, over the hill and far way.
  Mommy duck said, "Quack, quack, quack."
  And, 2 little ducks came waddling back.

- "A Hunting We Will Go"
  In this song, the refrain of the following is used each time:
  A hunting we will go. A hunting we will go.
  We'll catch a _____ and put him in a _____.
  A hunting we will go.

Table 3–2. Suggestions for Animal and Object Pairs for Rhyming Songs

Farm Animals	Woods/Forest Animals	Pets	Household Items	Clothing
goat/coat	fox/box	cat/hat	chair/bear	shirt/hurt
hen/pen	deer/gear	dog/log	couch/slouch	pants/ants
pig/wig	goose or moose/caboose	mouse/house	bed/red/said	shorts/ports
sheep/jeep	skunk/bunk	snake/lake	glass/bass	socks/rocks
lamb/jam	frog/log/jog	rat/pat/mat	plate/slate/skate	hat/mat/rat
cow/bow	raccoon/spoon/moon		spoon/moon	coat/moat
calf/half	dove/glove		room/boom	shoe/too
	bee/tree		rug/slug/mug	boot/root
	bear/care/fair		clock/rock	

Step 4: Use books that rhyme.

Many published books include rhymes. Dr. Seuss has many early readers that rhyme. There also are free Web sites such as http://www.hubbardscupboard.org and http://carlscorner.us.com that provide printable books with word family patterns (rhyming patterns). Parents and caregivers should be encouraged to read books that rhyme in order to increase familiarization with the pattern of rhyming words.

Strategy 2: Here's How to Introduce Phonological Awareness in a Sentence

Besides the ability to rhyme words, awareness of individual words and the ability to discriminate words in a sentence is another phonological awareness skill that is necessary for academic success. A child must understand that separate words make up a sentence before he or she will understand that sounds make up individual words.

Step 1: Introduce words that make up a sentence.

- Start with a simple sentence such as, "I go."
- The adult demonstrates a clap for each word.

clap	clap
I	go

- The preschooler or kindergarten student then claps with the adult.
- The adult introduces another two-word sentence slowly and pauses between the words and asks the student to provide the number of claps.
- The adult then introduces a three-word sentence and the student and adult clap together for each word.

Step 2: Introduce longer sentences (Table 3–3).

The adult should discuss words that have more than one syllable so the preschooler or kindergarten student understands that it is still one word regardless of how long the word is.

Strategy 3: Here's How to Introduce Awareness and Discrimination of Words Into Syllables

Once the child has figured out that words make up a sentence the child is then ready to understand that words may have one or several syllables. Books such as *40,000 Selected Words* provide numerous words with different syllables (Blockcolsky, Frazer, & Frazer, 1987).

Step 1: Separate words into syllables.

- Start with a simple one-syllable word such as "me."

- The adult demonstrates a clap for each syllable.

clap
me

- The preschooler or kindergarten student then claps with the adult.
- The adult introduces another one-syllable word and asks the student to provide the number of claps for the one-syllable word.
- The adult then introduces a two-syllable word and the student and adult clap together for each word.
  - Begin with compound words.
  - Move to two-syllable words.

Step 2: Introduce words with increasing number of syllables (Table 3–4).

Table 3–3. Sample Sentences for Words Within a Sentence

Two-Word Sentences	Three-Word Sentences	Four-Word Sentences
I go.	I will go.	I will go shopping.
See you.	We will run.	We will play outside.
I can.	I ran today.	I want a snack.
I will.	I ran yesterday.	Where is the car?
I play.	I am five.	I like center time.
We run.	You are fun.	It is circle time.
We jump.	Let's go home.	Let's run and play.

Table 3–4. Example of Syllables in Words

One Syllable	Two Syllables	Three Syllables	Four Syllables
me	outside	yesterday	introduction
we	inside	tomorrow	concentration
he	beside	Saturday	subtraction
she	parkway	calendar	paratrooper
be	behind	portable	periwinkle
tree	over	telescope	particular

Strategy 4: Here's How to Introduce Phonemic Awareness and the Alphabetic Principle

Phonemic awareness is the foundation for phonics. A preschooler or kindergarten student must be able to discriminate the individual sounds in a word before being able to associate the letter or letters with the sound. Once the student can associate the letter or letters with the sound, he or she is then ready to learn the phonics rules of the English language. Strategies for phonemic awareness provide opportunities to explore speech sounds with and without the letter association.

Step 1: Introduce letters, diagraphs, and diphthongs and their sounds (Table 3–5).

An alphabet chart or strip plus beginning consonant diagraphs (ch, sh, th) and diphthongs (oi/oy, ow/ou, au/aw, oo) can be used to associate a letter or set of letters with their speech sound. First, the speech-language pathologist or educator says the alphabet letter then provides a cue, as described next, that goes with the sound. For example, the cue for /b/ could be pretending to bounce a ball. So the speech-language pathologist or educator would say the letter "B" then provide the hand movement while making the /b/ sound. Each subsequent letter is stated the same way. Then the preschooler or kindergarten student also states the letter sound and imitates the hand movement while saying the sound. This will assist the student with hearing the sounds correctly and begin to start associating the letter that goes with the sound. Speech sounds should be kept as pure as possible. Do not add a schwa vowel after the sound (/b/ instead of /ba/). Preschool children with language difficulties often will have difficulty with beginning phonics and blending of sounds if a schwa vowel is added. They do not automatically learn to drop it off when attempting to use phonics for writing words.

The alphabet sound is said in the order of the alphabet song with additional diagraphs and diphthongs sounds given at the end. Additional sounds for letters such as soft /c/ and soft /g/ are introduced as the phonic rule /c/ or /g/ followed by /i/, /e/, or /y/ makes their soft sound /s/ as in city and /j/ as in gym. These visual and auditory cues allow the preschooler or kindergarten student to begin to understand the sounds. Because it has been introduced for speech production, the foundation is provided for phonemic and phonological awareness and for beginning phonics skills. As the preschooler or kindergarten student is attempting to sound out a word, the speech-language pathologist or teacher can use the hand signals to assist the student in the next sound. The student can also use the cue to recall or retrieve the letter associated with the sound.

Step 2: Locate the sound in a word using color cubes

This step in phonemic awareness requires the ability to understand beginning, middle, and end, thus further supporting sequencing strategies and understanding time/sequence concepts.

Table 3–5. Suggestions for Alphabet Sounds, Diagraphs, and Diphthongs

Letter	Suggestions for Visual Cue
a	Short vowel: Point to mouth and say /a/, /a/, /a/ Long vowel: Two thumbs up for /ae/
b	Action like bouncing a ball
c	Hard /c/: click of a camera
d	Action like beating a drum or raindrops dripping
e	Short vowel: Hands up to indicate "I don't know" and move head side to side Long vowel: Motion like a squeaky door opening
f	1. Action like a fish swimming 2. Cat hissing
g	Action like a monster saying /g/ or taking a big drink and swallowing
h	1. Wave hand in front of mouth like something is hot 2. dog panting
i	Short vowel: Rub thumb and index finger together like something is small Long vowel: Point to "eye"
j	1. Jump up and down while making the sound 2. Jumping rope
k	Kicking motion
l	1. Licking like a lollipop 2. Singing such as "la la la" (remember to keep sound pure /l/, /l/, /l/)
m	Rub belly and make sound for /m/ like it tastes good
n	Shake index finger as if stating "wrong choice"

Letter	Suggestions for Visual Cue
o	Short vowel: 1. Place hands joined above head and say sound 2. Move hands like an octopus Long vowel: Place hand over mouth like surprised /oh/
p	1. Move hands in front of body like pushing something 2. Open and close fingers like popcorn popping
q	Pretend to be putting on a king's or queen's crown (kw)
r	1. Pretend to be running 2. Dog growling
s	Move index forward like a snake while making the /s/ sound
t	Rub index fingers together to indicate tsk tsk
u	Short vowel: Pretend to pull a rope Long vowel: Point to other person, indicating "you"
v	Move hands up to make a /v/ like victory
w	1. Move hand like washing a window 2. Baby crying
x	1. Bacon in a frying pan and make the pan move while making /ks/ 2. Move fingers down like sprinkling water on a hot pan
y	Motion like playing with a yoyo
z	1. Bee buzzing 2. Zipper zipping
ch	Move arm like pulling the bell on a train /ch/ /ch/

continues

Table 3–5. *continued*

Letter	Suggestions for Visual Cue
sh	Finger in front of mouth like "be quiet"
th	Unvoiced: Act like opening a beach ball and the air coming out
th	Voiced: Move hand like sawing and make the /th/ sound
oi/oy	Make a pig noise while moving hand as if going down a slide

Letter	Suggestions for Visual Cue
oo	oo (boot): Make a noise like something is really neat (oooooooo)
	oo (foot): Make a noise like a car trying to start
au/aw	Cover mouth as if yawning while making the sound
ou/ow	Pinch own arm while saying /ow/

Note: From Margo Kinzer Courter, MBA, MA, CCC-SLP, Courter Communications, LLC.

- One-inch cubes of different colors (these can be purchased online by placing "1-inch plastic cubes" in the search engine) are used to represent speech sounds. Each color represents one sound. If the same sound is present in the same word, then the same color block is used.

- The speech-language pathologist presents a sound for which the preschooler or kindergarten student should listen.

- Then the speech-language pathologist or educator presents the sounds of the word while pointing to the corresponding block in the following order:

  1. Consonant-vowel (CV) or vowel-consonant (VC).
  2. Consonant-short vowel-consonant (CVC) words.
  3. Consonant-long vowel-consonant (CVCe). Remember that this still is presented with three blocks because the blocks are based on sound, not letters in the word.
  4. Consonant 1-consonant 2-vowel-consonant (beginning blends).

- The student is asked to point to one of the sounds presented.

- Then the student points to the cube that corresponds to the sound presented as the target sound.

- The student states where the sound is located. This would be the beginning, middle, or end of the word or first, second, third, fourth, and so on.

Block example (different colors would be used to represent each different sound):

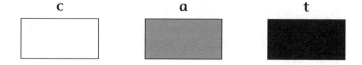

Steps in the block example:

The speech-language pathologist or educator:

1. places blocks in a row to indicate each speech sound in the word
2. states for the preschooler or kindergarten student to listen for the /a/ sound
3. says each sound (purely) as each block is touched

The preschooler or kindergarten student:

4. touches the block that designates the sound stated
5. states if the sound is in the beginning, middle, or end of the word based on the location of the block chosen

Please remember that this is based on pure sounds, not letters. For example, /sh/, /th/, /ch/ are one sound but two letters. While working with the blocks, this is presented with one block because it is one sound. Long vowel words also are presented with the number of sounds in the word, not how many letters they represent. These can be described as phonic rules later by stating that two letters make one sound. "What two letters go together to make /sh/?" or "The vowel sound is 'name.' So, who do you think will be the helper?" Remember: "Old Mac-Donald had a vowel a, e, i, o, u . . . and sometimes y."

Strategy 5: Here's How to Use Programs for Individuals and Groups

If a preschooler or kindergarten student continues to demonstrate difficulty with phonemic and phonological awareness, a more structured approach may be needed in therapy or in the classroom. The speech-language pathologist can be instrumental as part of a team choosing a program or assisting in devising a program based on the state's educational standards for preschool or kindergarten.

Programs should be research based with a structured approach to teaching phonological awareness, phonics, whole words, and beginning reading and writing. Programs such as the Letter People (Friedmann & Reiss-Weimann, 2009) and Road to the Code (Blachman, Ball, Black, & Tangel, 2000) are research-based programs that could be considered when assisting a classroom in choosing a program.

Narrative Skills Introduction

As stated in the introduction, a child's narrative skills provides a window into his or her language comprehension, command of vocabulary, and expression. The child demonstrates his or her vocabulary knowledge, concept development, sequencing abilities, ability to formulate grammatically correct sentences in addition to developing critical thinking (making predictions and inferences). We also can assess the complexity of the sentences being used during narration. In addition, the child can demonstrate verbal turn taking and participating in a discussion of the story. The adult can use a story in order to embed other skills such as phonological awareness skills, listening skills, and further concept and vocabulary development.

Area: Narrative Skills

Examples of Goals

The preschooler or kindergarten student will:

1. increase the ability to accurately sequence the events in a story
2. increase the ability to use vocabulary appropriate for the story
3. demonstrate comprehension of the story
4. demonstrate knowledge of the concepts presented (e.g., before, after, during, in, out, over, etc.) in printed materials as well as the specific story
5. make predictions and inferences regarding the story
6. use grammatically correct sentences in the story retell

Rationale: Narrative skills rely on language comprehension, command of vocabulary, and oral expression. Much information can be gathered from analyzing a child's ability to retell stories.

Developing Narrative Skills Strategies

There are many creative ways to use children's books to increase all of the areas needed for excellent narrative skills.

Listening Skills: By having the child actively participate in the telling of a story, the child will be listening more attentively for when they are called on for participation. For example, if the class is acting out the "Three Little Pigs," and one child is the Big Bad Wolf, he or she will need to pay closer attention to when the Big Bad Wolf is presented in the story.

Listening Comprehension: After a story is told, the storyteller can ask questions to assess the children's comprehension of the story.

Critical Thinking: The storyteller also can ask questions during the story about what will happen next. Questions can be asked regarding why parts of the story occurred the way they did. If there are several versions of a story, conversations can occur regarding the various endings.

Auditory Short-Term Memory: The storyteller can ask the children to repeat key phrases or repetitive verses in the story.

Concept Development: Printed stories allow development of spatial concepts such as front, back, middle, top, bottom. Story retell develops concepts of color/shape, time, quantity, location, condition, quality, and emotions.

Sequencing: As the child retells the story, the ability to sequence information develops. This also would include time concepts such as beginning, middle, end, first, and last.

Vocabulary: By choosing specific vocabulary from a story, the adult can work on developing vocabulary skills such as knowledge of the words in the stories as well as synonyms and antonyms for those words.

Sentence Formulation: As the child develops narrative skills, concepts, and vocabulary, these skills can be used to formulate more sophisticated sentences (adjectives, adverbs, compound sentences, complex sentences).

Phonological Awareness: The storyteller also can develop phonological awareness skills while working on narrative skills. This may include syllables in a sentence; syllables in words; beginning, middle, and ending sounds; and rhyming words.

Verbal Turn Taking: Pragmatically, narrative skills allow a child to discuss a story rather than only retelling a story.

A child's narrative skills and narrative development are critical to future academic success. It is amazing how many language skills are necessary and can be developed through this process.

In conclusion, speech-language pathologists and educators can see patterns of learning emerge with very young preschool children. Preschool children who are demonstrating difficulty following auditory directions or repeating words or sentences verbatim may have signs of auditory short-term memory difficulties. Preschool children who have difficulty with delayed expressive vocabulary may be demonstrating signs of word-finding difficulties. Preschool children with voicing and vowel distortions may demonstrate difficulty later with perceiving spoken words correctly, thus difficulty with multimeaning of words. These same preschooler or kindergarten students may demonstrate difficulty with perceiving sounds correctly in spoken words owing to their own perceptual errors, thus later difficulty with phonological awareness activities due to misperception of sounds. A child's narrative skills also provide a glimpse of all of the preceding skills during a single activity. It is vital to understand how speech and language difficulties of preschool children may impact later literacy and academic success.

The following summary is provided as a quick reference while treating preschool children.

Preschool Language Skills and Possible Academic Effects

Many receptive (understanding) and expressive (talking) milestones for young children are very important for later learning success. Difficulty in mastering these skills may be indicative of underlying speech and/or language difficulties that could affect learning as the child enters and progresses through school. Table 3–6 shows language milestones and how they may affect future learning.

Table 3–6. Language Milestones and Effects on Future Learning

Language Skills	What Could It Mean?
Late Talker	Research shows that children who are late talkers are at greater risk for academic difficulties, especially in literacy and reading skills.
Following Directions, Repeating Sentences, Songs, Nursery Rhymes, Prayers	The ability to follow directions of increasing complexity (one step, two step related, two step unrelated, etc.) and the ability to repeat information verbatim may be indicative of difficulty with auditory short-term memory (short-term memory). Good auditory short-term memory is needed in the classroom in order to follow the teacher's directions, remember to bring books and assignments home, and hold onto the teacher's explanations or lectures in order to take notes.
Understanding Rhymes	This is a preliteracy skill (phonological awareness) that assists with understanding onset and rimes (word families such as at, cat, hat, bat, sat), which assists with identifying patterns, chunking, and segmenting for spelling and reading easier.
Produce Members in a Category (Rapid Automatic Naming), Expressing Colors, and Shapes	Difficulty with these skills may be indicative of a word finding problem. Children with word finding disorders have difficulty recalling colors, shapes, alphabet letters, sounds of the alphabet letters for beginning phonics, and recalling sight words even though they know the information. This leads to guessing at words. Sometimes the words recalled will be wrong, which will affect comprehension.
Vocabulary Skills	A decrease in understanding and producing vocabulary will make increasing vocabulary skills for school-related topics difficult.
Sequencing	Sequencing begins with understanding first and last as well as the use of past tense verbs (to understand sequence of past events) and future tense verbs (to understand what will occur). Children need to be able to understand sequencing words. They should be able to sequence in order to sequence stories that they hear and read. This also leads to understanding the main idea of the story and the details that support the main idea.
Narrative Skills	A decrease in narrative skills has major implications for future learning. The ability to retell a story includes auditory comprehension of the story, oral expression, vocabulary, sequencing, sentence formulation, memory, and critical thinking.

Conclusion

In summary, even if speech-language pathologists or educators are working with preschool children, we need to monitor acquisition of developmental milestones closely. In addition, we need to be mindful of the developmental speech and language areas that could have an impact on literacy and future learning. Certain missing skills may be those that are very important for emerging literacy skills and overall academic success.

References

Blachman, B. A., Ball, E. W., Black, R., & Tangel, D. M. (2000). *Road to the code.* Baltimore, MD: Brookes.

Blockcolsky, V. D., Frazer, D. H., & Frazer, J. M. (1987). *40,000 selected words.* San Antonio, TX: Communication Skill Builders.

Bradley, L., & Bryant, P. (1983). Categorizing sounds and learning to read—A causal connection. *Nature, 301,* 419–421.

Childhood Apraxia of Speech Association. (n.d.). *Education related experiences and children with apraxia.* Retrieved September 7, 2009, from http://www.apraxia-kids.org

DeGaetano, J. G. (1994). *Processing auditory messages, exactly and totally.* Wrightsville Beach, NC: Great Ideas for Teaching.

Dickinson, D., & Tabors, P. (2001). *Beginning literacy with language.* Baltimore, MD: Brookes.

Do to Learn. (n.d.). Make a Schedule [Computer program]. Retrieved February 25, 2009, from http://www.dotolearn.com

Friedman, R., & Reiss-Weimann, E. (2009). Letter people. *Abrams Learning Trends, your resource for Early Childhood, Early Learning, Elementary Education.* Retrieved August 9, 2009, from http://www.abramslearningtrends.com

Hughes, D., McGillivray, L, & Schmidek, M. (1997). Guide to narrative language. Eau Claire, WI: Thinking Publications.

KIDiddles. (n.d.). *Children's songs with free lyrics, music and printable.* Retrieved March 1, 2009, from http://www.kididdles.com/

Lundberg, I., Olofsson, A., & Wall, S. (1980). Reading and spelling skills in the first years predicted from phonemic awareness skills in kindergarten. *Scandinavian Journal of Psychology, 21,* 159–173.

Mayer-Johnson. (n.d.). Board Maker [Computer program]. Retrieved February 25, 2009, from http://www.mayer-johnson.com

McGregor, K. (1997). The nature of word-finding errors of preschoolers with and without word-finding deficits. *Journal of Speech, Language, and Hearing Research, 40,* 1232–1244.

PBS Kids. (n.d.). *Barney and friends.* Retrieved March 1, 2009, from http://www.pbskids.org/barney

Reed, V. (2005). *An introduction to children with language disorders* (3rd ed.). Boston, MA: Pearson/Allyn and Bacon.

Rossetti, L. (1990). *Rossetti Infant Toddler Language Scale.* East Moline, IL: LinguiSystems.

Sharma, R., Purdy, S., & Kelly, A. (2009). Comorbidity of auditory processing, language, and reading disorders. *Journal of Speech, Language, and Hearing Research, 52,* 706–722.

Snow, C. E., Tabors, P. O., Nicholson, P., & Kurland, B. (1995). Oral language and early literacy skills in kindergarten and first grade children. *Journal of Research in Childhood Education, 10,* 37–48.

Therasimplicity. (n.d.). Sound Mapping [Computer program]. Retrieved February 22, 2009, from http://www.therasimplicity.com

Torgesen, J., Wagner, R., & Rashotte, C. (1994). Longitudinal studies of phonological processing and reading. *Journal of Learning Disabilities, 27,* 276–286.

Wilcox, M., Cheslock, M., Crais, E., Norman-Murch, T., Paul, R., & Roth, F. (2008). *Roles and responsibilities of speech-language pathologist in early intervention: Guidelines.* Rockville, MD: American Speech-Language-Hearing Association.

Zimmerman, I. L., Steiner, V. G., & Pond, R. E. (2002). *Preschool Language Scale 4 (PLS 4).* San Antonio, TX: Psychological Corporation.

4

Reading Is Rocket Science

Introduction

Educators often say that kindergarten through second grade students are learning to read and that students from third grade forward are reading to learn. This includes longer and more complex reading passages, increased critical thinking, as well as an increase on other subjects such as science and social studies. This has great significance for those students who are not demonstrating age-appropriate reading skills and reading comprehension by third grade. It has been my experience that a child has to be ready to enter kindergarten with mastery of many phonological awareness skills so that reading can occur early during the school year. A large body of research has linked deficient phonological awareness, specifically phonemic awareness, in kindergarten and the early grades with poor reading achievement (Blachman & Tangel, 2008). In chapter 2, Torgesen, Wagner, and Rashotte (1997) reported that children who began first grade with phonological awareness skills below the 20th percentile lagged behind their peers in word identification and word decoding throughout elementary school.

Reading instruction has changed over the years and continues to change based on the theories and research at the time. The Eunice Kennedy Shriner National Institute of Student Health and Human Development (2010) provides a framework for early reading practices to reduce reading difficulties. These include phonemic awareness, the alphabetic principle, decoding, word recognition skills, and use context to confirm understanding. Further research (Adams, 1994; Blachman & Tangel, 2008; Wylie & Durell, 1970) also supports the use of phonics based + whole word reading instruction for teaching reading.

The goal with working with any student with a speech or language disorder is to make sure that he or she will be successful in the daily environment, which means success in school. Speech-language pathologists are encouraged to address word finding; receptive and expressive language skills, including morphology, phonology, semantics, syntax, and pragmatics; as well as speech disorders through strategies that will increase success in learning to read. Success in learning to read and becoming a proficient reader will then lead to success throughout all academic areas. For many students with speech and language disorders, reading really is rocket science with complicated letters, sounds, and patterns. This chapter addresses strategies for early reading skills, reading accuracy, fluency, and reading comprehension.

Early Reading Introduction

Of children with language impairments, 40% to 65% may be diagnosed in the early grades with a reading disability (Catts, Fey, Tomblin, & Zhang, 2002). As stated in the introduction of this chapter, early reading skills, including phonological awareness, are critical to literacy success and overall academic success.

Area: Early Reading

Example of Goals

The student will increase:

1. phonological awareness skills
2.   understanding and production of closed syllables (consonant-vowel-consonant)
3. retrieval skills for whole words and word families

Rationale: As stated, students with speech and language difficulties often demonstrate difficulty with beginning reading skills. The preceding goals will assist the beginning reader in making the connection between letters and sounds introduced before this time with beginning reading.

Early Reading Strategies

Strategy 1: Here's How to Improve Onset and Rime for Word Family Recognition

I have seen the moment many times when a younger child finally figures out rhyming words. Initially, the child will demonstrate an inability or reluctance to participate in songs and finger plays. With adapting materials in therapy, the child begins to perceive the rhyming involved and will then begin to enjoy the songs. Once the student is able to perceive rhyming patterns correctly, word families can be introduced so that he or she can see the pattern emerge.

Because of the amount of information that the early reader is attempting to learn, introducing the letters that represent word families adds one more component. Initially, the speech-language pathologist or educator is encouraged to use patterns (consonant-vowel) that are actual words that the student will learn when learning high-frequency words so they are linked to the whole words that he or she is learning. This includes words such as "in," "an," "it," "at," and "up." After the student begins to understand these segments, other word families can be added. It is my experience that this will make segmenting multisyllable words easier as they are introduced.

Chapter 3 targets block work for discrimination of each sound in a simple word. In this activity, two blocks are kept together to demonstrate to the child that a word family stays together and only the first sound changes (Table 4–1).

This task can be introduced to prekindergarten children without introducing the letter/sound association. As the child begins to learn letter/sound association, the letters can be added to show that many times word families are spelled the same. As stated previously, this task can begin with using high-frequency words that the student is learning (and, up, at, it, in).

Strategy 2: Here's How to Introduce Phonics and the Alphabetic Principle

In chapter 3, the alphabet, diphthongs, and digraphs were introduced with the speech-language pathologist or the educator stating each letter with a hand signal to link the sound with the letter. The speech-language pathologist or educator can now use cubes and the hand signals to assist the student with hearing each sound accurately and begin to blend these together.

The alphabetic principle: The systematic and predictable relationship between written letters and spoken sounds.

Table 4–1. Block Examples

c	a	t

b	a	t

m	a	t

> **Diphthong:** Two vowel sounds produced together (e.g., au, aw, oi, oy, ou, ow).

> **Digraph:** A pair of letters representing a single sound (e.g., /ph/, /ch/, /sh/, /th/).

Step 1: Use blocks to represent sounds.

This activity combines phonological awareness of identification of individual sounds in words and the ability to manipulate the order of the sounds and changes in the sounds within the word. In addition it brings in the idea that the sounds are represented by a letter or combination of letters (alphabetic principle). The speech-language pathologist or educator will place three blocks on the table. A different color should be used for each sound. If the sound is the same, the same color block is used. So, if the word "cat" is the chosen word, three blocks of different colors would be placed on the table. For example, a red block could represent /c/, a blue block to represent /a/, and a yellow block to represent /t/. If the word was "bib," two of the same color block would be placed on the table because there are two sounds that are the same. A second color block would be used for /i/.

Step 2: Use pictures for consonant-vowel-consonant words.

Present a picture that represents a consonant-vowel-consonant (CVC) word (also referred to as a closed syllable word) so that the student can see the picture, say the word, and use blocks to represent each sound. If the words are presented in the order listed in Table 4–2, the student will begin to see the pattern of onset and

Table 4–2. CVC Pictures/Words Examples

bat	jet	fog	pig	mop	man
cat	pet	dog	big	top	pan
hat	wet	log	wig	pop	can
fat	cap	hog	cup	hop	tan
mat	map	red	pup	sit	van
rat	gap	bed	tub	hit	ran
sat	lap	fed	cub	lit	fan
pat	nap	wed	rub	pit	ban

rimes work with letters because only the first letter/sound changes. During this activity, the blocks should not be placed together to represent the word family as in Strategy 1. The goal is for the student to demonstrate correct discrimination and perception of each sound individually in order to use individual sounds to form words.

Step 3: Change the pattern.

Once the student is successful with CVC words, the pattern can change. This would include consonant-vowel-consonant-consonant (CVCC) words and consonant-consonant-vowel-consonant (CCVC) words (Table 4–3). This step introduces initial and final blends and endings such as -ing.

With this task, the student can begin to see patterns in words. For example, once he or she learns -ing and -er, it is easier to chunk these segments in order to decode or encode the word.

Strategy 3: Here's How to Introduce Phonetically Regular Words

A phonetically regular word is a word that has a common phoneme-grapheme relationship and can be sounded out (decoded). This applies to one-syllable words as well as multisyllable words.

Step 1: Present phonetically regular words.

Present phonetically regular words orally for the student to use blocks in order to write the words. Phonetically regular words are words that follow the sounds usually represented by the consonants or vowels. These words also would include digraphs and diphthongs (Table 4–4).

Step 2: Maintain the same pattern.

Words can be presented following the same word family so that the student can discriminate the rhyming pattern and would only change the first sound.

Step 3: Change the pattern with each new word.

Words that would change the entire word pattern each time also can be presented. For example, the word "cat" may be presented. The second word may be "pig," which would represent a different sound pattern.

Table 4–3. CVCC and CCVC Pictures/Words Examples

band	sing	glad	spit	flop	flip
hand	ring	flap	slit	plop	clip
land	ding	clap	plan	stop	slip
sand	ping		clan		

Table 4–4. Phonetically Regular Words

at	ad	ap	al	am	an	ab	ag
bat	bad	cap	gal	bam	ban	cab	bag
fat	cad	gap	pal	dam	can	fab	gag
hat	fad	lap		ham	Dan	lab	lag
mat	mad	map		Pam	fan	tab	nag
pat	pad	nap		ram	man		rag
rat	sad	rap		Sam	pan		sag
sat		sap			ran		tag
		tap			tan		

it	in	id	ib	ig	im	ip	ed
bit	bin	bid	bib	big	dim	dip	bed
fit	fin	hid	fib	dig	rim	hip	fed
hit	pin	lid	rib	fig	Tim	lip	led
lit		rid		jig		rip	ted
pit				pig		sip	wed
sit				rig		tip	
kit				wig			
wit							

en	et	ob	ot	op	od	og	ug
den	bet	cob	cot	bop	cod	bog	bug
hen	get	rob	got	cop	nod	cog	hug
men	jet		hot	hop	pod	dog	jug
pen	let		not	pop	rod	fog	mug
ten	met		pot	top	sod	hog	rug
	pet		rot			log	tug
	set		tot				

ub	un
cub	bun
hub	fun
rub	gun
tub	pun
	run
	sun

Strategy 4: Here's How to Use Fun Activities to Practice Rhyming and Phonetically Regular Words

Activity 1: Adapting materials for songs and finger plays

Obtain adaptive books or pictures for songs and finger plays that can be used with Velcro or magnets on a board. This gives the student the opportunity to manipulate the objects while learning the patterns of the songs or finger plays.

Step 1: Find or make pictures.
Find or make pictures (with cardstock and a laminator) to represent songs and finger plays.

Step 2: Write the words on the pictures.
A permanent marker or label maker works great for materials that are already laminated. If the educator is making the materials, the words can be written before the picture is laminated in order to better preserve the letters.

Step 3: Assist with seeing the words and word patterns.
As the student manipulates the pictures, he or she will see the words and word patterns that represent those words.

Activity 2: Playing ball

Use a ready-made ball such as Clever Catch Balls by American Educational Products (n.d.) or take a soccer or beach ball and make a ball that has phonetically regular words.

Step 1: Ask the student to express where his or her left thumb is.

Step 2: When the student catches the ball, the word that the left thumb landed on is the word that the student says.

Activity 3: If you can spell . . .

This activity can be performed when throwing a ball back and forth or swinging on a swing or verbally without a play activity. (This also is a great car game that parents can play with their student.)

Step 1: Give the student a word to spell, such as "at."

Step 2: After the student spells the word, state, "If you can spell _____, you can spell _____." For example, "If you can spell at, you can spell cat."

Step 3: Continue playing the game until the student misspells the word.

Step 4: Change the pattern when the student misspells the word.

These games can be adapted for high-frequency word practice.

Strategy 5: Here's How to Introduce Crucial Phonics Rule

There are programs, such as Road to Reading, that are based on understanding the crucial components that research has shown to be necessary to be a successful reader (Blachman & Tangel, 2008). Another program that is used in many schools, at least in my geographical area, is VOWAC. VOWAC refers to the following components for teaching vowel patterns as the CLOVER method. These include:

- Closed Syllables. For closed syllables, the student is introduced to CVC words and the consonant digraphs for /ck/, /ch/, /sh/, and /th/.
- Final e. The rule of the final /e/ is introduced. This letter as the final sound is often referred to as magic /e/ or helper /e/.
- Open syllable. CV words are introduced where the vowel makes the long sound (he, me, we, she) and CV syllables that make the long sound (si-lent).
- Vowel teams. This rule addresses two vowels together. The saying that goes with vowel teams that represent the long vowel sound is that when two vowels go walking, the first one does the talking. This level also introduces the diphthongs /oi/, /oy/, /ow/, /ou/, /au/, and /aw/.
- Vowel + /r/. This rule includes /ur/, /ir/, /er/, /or/, and /ar/. Other sounds for vowel + /r/ (ere, air, ear) can be introduced at a later time.
- Consonants + /le/. The suffix /le/ is introduced with the consonants that can accompany it (VoWac Publishing Co., n.d.)

Using a structured program, such as Road to Reading or VOWAC, provides many advantages, including a structure for all educators to be on the same page while working with the same students; a framework for discussion among professionals regarding a student's reading progress; and a systematic approach to assist the struggling reader. This keeps the educator from moving too far ahead too fast.

Strategy 6: Here's How to Introduce High-Frequency Words

As discussed earlier, a multilevel approach is necessary for children with a speech and/or language disorder with comorbid learning and reading disorders. The ability of these students to recognize and produce high-frequency words accurately will increase their reading accuracy and fluency rate. For students with a word-finding disorder, frequent practice of the high-frequency words is important in order for them to recall the word accurately. Speech-language pathologists and educators need to remember that words should be linked to both their semantic meaning and ways to increase the retrieval strength. Students with a word-finding disorder often state the first word that they are able to retrieve that starts with the same letter (perceptual/visual error) as the word in text. This leads to reading comprehension difficulties because of misreading the word. The student may read, "The house runs." But the statement should have been, "The horse runs." Often, the child will continue to read and not question the accuracy of what was read. It is therefore easy to understand how this will lead to reading comprehension difficulties.

Activity 1: Using picture cards or computer software to link high-frequency words with their meaning (and retrieval strength)

Present pictures with the word that represents the picture on the same card or on the opposite side. This will provide meaning to the words. This can be accomplished with ready-made pictures that pair the word with the picture, or as described previously in the fun activities the speech-language pathologist or educator can add the words with a permanent marker to already made materials or to materials that are made. Pictures can be obtained through picture programs such as Mayer-Johnson Boardmaker (2006–2010), Do To Learn pictures (n.d.), Therasimplicity (n.d.), Google images (n.d.), or other computer-based programs.

There also are computer programs, such as Mayer-Johnson Writing with Symbols (2000), that provide a picture to represent words. This type of program allows a student to look at a storybook and sequence the story in the student's own words. The speech-language pathologist or educator can type what the student says, or the older student can type and practice keyboarding skills at the same time. The story can then be printed so that the student can use the pictures to recall the story and the words represented by the pictures. This will increase the link between the high-frequency word and the picture that it represents because the student will see the same word with the same picture each time (Mayer-Johnson, 2000).

Activity 2: Memorizing and recalling high-frequency words

A strategy to learn and recall high-frequency words is presented in chapter 5 in more depth. This includes using modeling clay to represent the meaning of the word (Davis, 1994). A picture that represents what was made can be placed on the back of the index card. This should be a picture of the meaning, not a picture of a sentence where the word is used. For students with a word-finding disorder, a strategy to increase retrieval strength also needs to be added to the index card. The strategy used will be based on the error pattern type presented. Students with word-finding difficulties need to review the high-frequency words frequently in order to assist with recall. "Frequently" means at least daily if not several times a day. Once it appears that the student can always recall the word, the next group of words should be targeted. The previous words then need to be presented again to ensure that the word has been moved to long-term memory and can be retrieved easily. The earlier groups can be added to the new words.

Activity 3: Using Elkonin boxes

Elkonin boxes also can be used to provide a visual representation for the letters (Griffith & Olson, 1992). An Elkonin box is a grid into which the letters fit to represent the word. The boxes are either square or rectangular to represent if the word stays between the dotted and the bottom solid lines on primary paper (square) or if the word goes above or below the lines (Table 4–5).

Using Elkonin boxes also will assist the student in understanding the printed letters and words and left-to-right progression and how to make the printed letters correctly.

Table 4–5. Examples of Elkonin Boxes

s	u	n

| t | a | g |

| b | e | d |

Activity 4: Learning high-frequency words

High-frequency words have a variety of names depending on the school that the student attends. These often are called *wall words*, *sight words*, *red words*, or *challenge words*. Simply, they are the most frequently used words in the English language. By learning high-frequency words, a student is able to read more fluently and accurately. The high-frequency words that are recalled/retrieved consistently also can be placed in phrases so that the student can begin to recognize these words surrounded by other words. Dolch word lists, Houghton Mifflin High Frequency Words, National Reading Vocabulary, Enchanted Learning, or other word lists can be used. As noted earlier, children with language disorders that affect learning may have difficulty recognizing the single word when it is placed with other words. They may attempt to revert to old habits and guess the word by quickly recalling a word that starts with the same letter.

Strategy 7: Here's How to Use Books With High-Frequency and Phonetically Regular Words

Books can be introduced after the student understands phonics and phonetically regular words and has learned several high-frequency words and word family groups. Many book series are available commercially for beginning reading. These include Reading A–Z, Scholastic Leveled Readers, Leveled Reader.com, and I Can Read books. Typically, these are labeled either by numbers (I, II, III) or by letters (A–Z) with the more simplistic books being Level I or A. There also are online sites such as Hubbard's Cupboard or Carl's Corner (n.d.) that provide printable high-frequency word and word family books for educators.

Building Reading Success Introduction

Once the student begins to demonstrate success with sounding out words and recalling high-frequency words, reading begins. Success with leveled readers is the next step. As the student is ready to tackle more difficult words and reading materials, successful reading habits have begun.

Area: Building Reading Success

Example of Goals

The student will increase:

1. reading accuracy
2. reading fluency
3. the ability to segment multisyllable words
4. encoding skills
5. decoding skills

Rationale: Once the student begins to read, he or she is not out of the woods yet. According to the 2007 National Assessment of Educational Progress, only 67% of the nation's fourth graders read at a basic level for their grade level. The basic level requires students to demonstrate an understanding of the overall meaning of what is read; that is, they can make connections between the text and their own experiences and make simple inferences. This study has significance for children who struggle to learn to read in early elementary school. They may continue to demonstrate difficulty with reading at their expected grade level when reading should be used for learning (National Assessment of Educational Progress, 2007). As demonstrated in this report, reading fluency, accuracy, and comprehension often continue to require intervention in order for the older student to at least reach the basic reading requirements.

Building Reading Success Strategies

Strategy 1: Here's How to Segment Multisyllable Words

Students often look at a multisyllable word and automatically state that they cannot read the word. Once they are shown that a multisyllable word is often just a long word made up of little words (compound words), word families, prefixes, or suffixes, they realize that they can segment the word and figure it out.

Activity 1: Teaching syllabification rules

- Syllables are chunks of sounds in a word that are produced in one breath.

- Each syllable contains at least a vowel. It might include a consonant but does not need to.

- Often affixes (prefixes and suffixes) are part of the word.

- One-syllable word families or high-frequency words often are part of the word.

- Look for syllable patterns (closed and open syllables, final /e/, vowel teams, vowel+/r/, and -le).

Activity 2: Introducing affixes and their meaning

The most frequently used prefixes (dis, un, mis, anti, de, inter, intra) should be introduced with their meaning. The most frequently used suffixes (-able, -ible, -le, -al, tion, ation) and their meaning should be introduced. These can be presented on cards, such as the ones that are discussed in chapter 5, for vocabulary words. The affix would go on the front of the tent card in place of the vocabulary word and the definition would be written on the inside lower section of the card.

Activity 3: Practicing each syllable in isolation

During this activity, the student is shown each syllable separately. He or she should produce the syllables in isolation, concentrating on affixes and syllable rules.

Activity 4: Decoding chunks

Step 1: Give the written multisyllable word, separated into the syllables, for the student to blend together. These can be written on index cards or by using syllable tiles that can be purchased at a teacher's store or online such as http://www.primary concepts.com.

Step 2: Present the words as a whole. The student then circles the syllabification rules. Once successful identifying the parts, the student is encouraged to sound out each syllable and blend the word. There are games such as Syllabification or syllable tiles that can be used for this step.

Activity 5: Spelling multisyllable words

Step 1: Have the student use blocks to represent each syllable that was heard. The student then touches the block as the syllable is written.

Step 2: Ask the student to tap down his or her arm to represent each syllable to understand how many parts of the word he or she has to write.

Strategy 2: Here's How to Increase Reading Accuracy

Many students with reading disorders often learn some high-frequency words and attempt to apply these words when reading, especially when they see another word in print that starts with the same letter as a high-frequency word they know. For example, the student sees the word "card" while reading and substitutes the word "car." This then changes the context of the sentence, thus the ability to correctly understand the sentence. The sentence states, "The card is turned over." The student then reads, "The car is turned over." If this sentence is presented as part of a paragraph, the meaning of the paragraph would change. Due to ongoing development of critical thinking and reading comprehension, the student may not realize that the sentence does not make sense even in the context of the other sentences in the paragraph. One can see how this affects reading accuracy, thus reading comprehension. Learning as many high-frequency words as possible, recognizing word families, and using phonics rules as needed will make the student a faster and more accurate reader.

Students with a reading disability often become overwhelmed quickly due to the number of words on the page. Accuracy then decreases further because of the increased demands. Many strategies are available to decrease the students' stress in reading while increasing reading accuracy.

Activity 1: Using a reading strip

Reading strips that highlight the current row works well for these students. They reduce the visual stimulation on the page. These can be purchased commercially or can be made by using two strips of card stock and packing tape. The strips are placed the distance apart that will allow the sentence to be viewed in the open area. This distance will depend on the size of print. Packing tape can then be placed to a join the card stock together.

Activity 2: Using an index card

Using an index card to block the sentences that have not been read takes away the visual overstimulation of the page. Care should be given to not cover pictures that may assist with figuring out unknown or difficult-to-retrieve words. The pictures will also assist with comprehension of the words on the page.

Activity 3: Using guided oral reading

The following steps can be used to assist with increasing reading fluency and accuracy:

1. The adult reads a passage aloud that is at the student's level.
2. The student rereads the passage silently at least once.
3. Then the passage is read aloud by the student.
4. The student rereads the passage aloud at least one more time.

Activity 4: Reading and rereading the same stories

Speech-language pathologists, reading specialists, teachers, and parents should encourage their student to read and reread favorite stories. This gives the student the opportunity to build words in the story as high-frequency words. It also increases fluency and reading comprehension. Many times, the student will memorize the story and need to be reminded to place a finger under each word so that the word is being visualized each time.

Activity 5: Using paired reading

Paired reading is accomplished by having two readers (Rasinski, 2003). The first reader is a skilled reader, such as a speech-language pathologist, an educator, or a parent. The second reader is the student. The two readers begin reading together. The adult reads slightly faster than the student. The student follows the text with a finger. If the student makes an error, the adult waits to see if the student corrects it. If not, the adult points to the word and corrects it. The reading continues. The student signals when ready to read solo.

Activity 5: Using recorded readings

There are many options for recorded reading. These can be obtained on audio CD or downloaded to an MP3. Again, the student is encouraged to use a finger to follow along with the text while listening. The student could also use this for paired reading.

Activity 6: Using choral reading

Choral reading occurs when more than one student read together (Rasinski, 2003). A variety of strategies are used in choral reading:

- Refrain choral reading occurs when one student reads most of the text and the rest chime in to read key or repeated segments.

- Line per student choral reading occurs when each student reads a line then the entire group reads the final lines together.

- Dialogue choral reading occurs usually in a play format where there are several characters and each student reads the character's lines.

Please note that if a student has a word-finding disorder, guided reading, paired reading, recording readings, or choral reading more than likely will not increase oral reading proficiency if retrieval strength is not targeted. Dr. German and Dr. Newman (2007) revealed a significant discrepancy between the oral and silent reading of the same words in children with word-finding difficulties. Oral reading accuracy was very low, but their accuracy jumped to 90% when the students were given the same words on a silent reading recognition task. That discrepancy points out that oral reading is not accurate for the student with word-finding difficulties.

Strategy 3: Here's How to Measure Reading Fluency

The ability to read accurately at an acceptable fluency rate, based on the student's grade level, leads to increased reading comprehension. The student who reads too slowly will have difficulty following the context of the information read. The following guidelines are offered as a reference for the number of words per minute that students should be able to read at different grade levels. Rasinski (2003, p. 80) offers guidelines for reading fluency in Table 4–6.

Table 4–6. Correct Number of Words per Minute

Grade Level	Target Number of Correct Words per Minute
Second half of first grade	60
Second grade	90
Third grade	100
Fourth grade	110
Fifth grade	120
Sixth Grade	140

Note. From *The Fluent Reader: Oral Reading Strategies for Building Word Recognition, Fluency, and Comprehension*, by T. V. Rasinski, 2003, New York: Scholastic.

The reading passage used to assess reading accuracy should be at the grade level expectation. The student is given a passage to read aloud at the grade level expectation. The examiner follows along with a copy of the passage. The examiner sets a stopwatch for 60 seconds. The student reads for 1 minute with the examiner marking misreading or errors. At the end of 1 minute, the number of words read is counted. The number of errors is subtracted from this number, which then gives the number of words read correctly in 1 minute. The following formula can be used to determine reading accuracy.

$$\frac{\text{Number of words read correctly}}{\text{Total number of words in the sample}} = \text{Reading accuracy for a 1-minute sample}$$

Another method of calculating is to allow the student to complete an entire passage. The examiner uses a stopwatch to determine the length of time needed to read the passage. The examiner counts the number of words read aloud with the number of errors subtracted. The following formula is used:

$$\frac{\text{Number of words read correctly}}{\text{Number of seconds to read}} \times 60 = \text{Reading rate in 1 minute}$$

Again, keep in mind that reading fluency is not a strong indicator of reading success for students with word-finding disorders. Reading level should be based on vocabulary and word knowledge and comprehension assessed nonverbally. This can be accomplished by having the student point to key vocabulary and information that answers comprehension questions (German, 2010).

Strategy 4: Here's How to Increase Reading Comprehension

Increased reading fluency and accuracy should lead to increased comprehension of what is read. Students with speech and language disorders may require specific strategies to increase comprehension.

Step 1: Use books with pictures and simple stories.

Beginning reading books typically have pictures that assist with telling the story. These pictures can be used to assist the student with understanding what each page is about. As the student increases reading skills, the pictures can assist with figuring out the words in the written information. These pictures also can assist in comprehending the story. The student can use the beginning reading book for the following tasks:

- Use the pictures to gain an understanding of what the book content.

- Read the words. If having difficulty recalling a high-frequency word or sounding out a novel word, rescanning the picture on the page often leads to producing a key word.

- Retell the story, if requested, by scanning what was read and using the pictures to increase sequencing of the story. This will demonstrate comprehension of what was read.

- Answer wh- questions that may require the student to look back through what was read to find the answer.

- Answer reasoning questions in order to problem solve possible solutions.

- Begin to learn about characters, settings, plots, conflict, and conflict resolution while reading simple picture books.

Step 2: Use books with increasing number of sentences per page.

Leveled readers increase the complexity of the words as well as the number of words and sentences on the page as the level is increased. If more than two or three sentences are on a page, a reading strip or an index card may be needed to block some of the sentences for the beginning reader so that the number of words is not overwhelming. Often, the student will just look at the page and state, "I can't read this." This occurs by the student being visually overstimulated by the number of words on the page before even looking at the complexity of the words or whether or not the words are familiar.

Step 3: Use leveled readers designed for students with reading difficulties.

Many books are available that have content that is appropriate for a student of a certain age but is written at an easier reading level. Many of these that are offered in a series also include a workbook for targeting comprehension of the information. High Noon Books offers a series of high-interest books at different levels of readability (Simms, n.d.). The workbooks that accompany this series are similar in style to a workbook that may be used in a classroom.

For students with a word-finding disorder, reading level should be based on comprehension in silent oral reading tasks and not the fluency and accuracy in oral reading tasks. Diane German (2010) suggests the following: (1) creating multiple choice reading questions; (2) using silent reading recognition tasks to check knowledge of word meanings (point to the word that means afraid [frightened], point to the word that means to go up in the air [jump]; (3) using silent reading recognition tasks to check the ability to draw inferences from read text (point to where in the sentence it indicates the character is sad, near a solution, etc.); (4) using silent reading recognition tasks to check the ability to decode specific words (point to *where*, point to *cocoon*); and (5) having students answer reading comprehension questions by numbering and highlighting where each question's answer is in the text.

Strategy 5: Here's How to Begin Encoding Skills

Step 1: Teach journaling.

Students also will need to be able to take decoding (reading) skills to encoding (spelling) skills. A student can begin in prekindergarten and kindergarten by learning to journal. The beginning journals will mostly consist of pictures to describe an event or a story. As the student begins to understand the alphabetic principle, words will begin to appear in the journal. This may start with the student placing his or her name on the top. The day of the week or date also can be added. The student may begin by copying this from the board. As he or she begins to learn phonics, phonetically regular words, and high-frequency words, beginning sentences will begin to emerge. This will be enhanced further from first grade on when the student begins to experience spelling tests, which will continue to increase the number of words that the student has for the journal. The teacher can begin to stretch the students by providing a specific topic or requiring a certain number of the spelling words or vocabulary words from a story to be included in the journal.

Step 2: Design spelling tests.

Spelling tests can be designed to include phonetically regular word (common phoneme-grapheme relationships and can be easily and accurately sounded out or decoded) and high-frequency words. The phonetically regular words assist the child with learning the phonics rules and spelling patterns. If spelling tests are used in prekindergarten and kindergarten, simple phonics rules should be introduced, such as short vowel sounds. For first grade, phonics rules should be presented with caution regarding how many rules are being presented. For example, the long /i/ sound can be spelled by /y/ in consonant vowel words (my), by adding a final /e/ (bite), or by /igh/ (light). All of these rules should not be presented in the same spelling test. Allow the student to master one or two of the rules before adding the other rules. If the students overall do not demonstrate mastery of the rule, the same rule should continue to be targeted until mastery is observed.

This may take several weeks of presenting words with the same phonics rule before a new rule is introduced. For older children, a phonics rule approach can continue for spelling. This should include more difficult patterns, such as /ind/, /igh/, and /dge/, in addition to prefixes and suffixes. The meaning of the prefixes and suffixes should be part of the lesson.

Step 3: Use dictation

Many children with language difficulties experience problems with dictated sentences. This requires many skills for the student. It requires good auditory short-term memory. This student needs to be able to hold the complete sentence into short-term auditory memory. He or she also needs to be able to perceive each word correctly in order to link the appropriate meaning to the sentence. This aids in the short-term recall of the sentence. The student then needs to retrieve the words and their correct spelling in a timely fashion in order to write the sentence.

Conclusion

All students benefit from an organized phonics program and a beginning reading program that provides experience with phonological awareness, the alphabetic principle, high-frequency words, phonetically regular words, decoding and encoding, and written expression. In addition, any exercises that can be added that will assist with correct discrimination and perception of sounds and words will help students to talk and spell with greater accuracy and to have a better understanding of words with multimeanings as they are introduced because they perceived the words or sounds correctly the first time.

Educators are encouraged to use phonetically regular words following the same phonics rule for spelling. Also, several high-frequency words can be added and identified as so. The pattern should be discussed with all of the students. The student with a speech or language difficulty who continues to struggle with onset and rime and phonetically regular words may not pick up on the pattern automatically unless it is pointed out during the review of the words. Words from the reading book used in the classroom can be used as vocabulary or spelling words, thus increasing comprehension of the story. These words can become the challenge words in the weekly spelling test. This provides a win-win situation for the students. They are learning phonics patterns to better their reading ability as well as building vocabulary skills and high-frequency word recognition.

A program that is well supported through researched strategies and an organized structured approach to phonics, spelling, reading, and reading fluency and accuracy will lead to greater reading comprehension and academic success. A strong program beginning in kindergarten and first grade will lead to greater success for all students long term. A student with a speech and/or language disorder can be a strong reader with a well-laid foundation.

References

Adams, M. J. (1994). *Beginning to read: Thinking and learning about print*. Cambridge, MA: MIT Press.

American Educational Products - Online Store. (n.d.). Clever Catch Balls. Retrieved July 2, 2009, from http://www.amep.com/

Blachman, B. A., M., D., & Tangel, P. (2008). *Road to reading: A program for preventing and remediating reading difficulties*. Baltimore, MD: Paul H. Brookes.

Carl's Corner.htm. (n.d.). Retrieved July 2, 2009, from http://www.carlscorner.us.com

Catts, H., Fey, M., Tomblin, J. B., & Zhang, X. (2002). A longitudinal investigation of reading outcomes in children with language impairments. *Journal of Speech, Language, and Hearing Research, 45*, 1142–1157.

Davis, R. (1994). *The gift of dyslexia*. New York, NY: Ability Workshop Press.

Do to Learn. (n.d.). Make a Schedule [Computer program]. Retrieved July 2, 2009, from http://dotolearn.com

Eunice Kennedy Shriver National Institute of Child Health and Human Development, NIH, DHHS. (2010). Developing early literacy: Report of the National Early Literacy Panel (NA). Washington, DC: U.S. Government Printing Office.

German, D. (2010). American Speech-Language-Hearing Association Division I List Serve. Rockville, MD: American Speech-Language-Hearing Association. Posted September, 4, 2010.

German, D., & Newman, R (2007). Oral reading skills of children with oral language (word-finding) difficulties. *Reading Psychology, 28*(5), 397–442.

Google Images. (n.d.). Retrieved July 2, 2009, from http://images.google.com

Griffith, P., & Olson, M. (1992). Phonemic awareness helps beginning readers break the code. *The Reading Teacher, 7*(45), 516–522.

Hubbard's Cupboard. (n.d.). *Literacy*. Retrieved July 2, 2009, from http://www.hubbardscupboard.org

I Can Read. (n.d.). Retrieved September 6, 2009, from http://www.icanread.com

Learning Materials. (n.d.). *Syllabification game*. Retrieved September 6, 2009, from http://www.learning-materials.com

Mayer-Johnson. (2000). Writing with Symbols [Computer program]. Retrieved July 2, 2009, from http://www.mayer-johnson.com

Mayer-Johnson. (2006–2010). Boardmaker v. 6 [Computer program]. Retrieved April 16, 2011, from http://www.mayer-johnson.com

National Assessment of Educational Progress (NAEP). (n.d.). *The nation's report card*. Retrieved July 2, 2009, from http://nces.ed.gov/nationsreportcard

Primary Concepts. (n.d.). *Build a bigger word letter tiles*. Retrieved September 6, 2009, from http://www.primaryconcepts.com

Rasinski, T. V. (2003). *The fluent reader: Oral reading strategies for building word recognition, fluency, and comprehension*. New York, NY: Scholastic.

Reading A-Z. (n.d.). Retrieved September 6, 2009, from http://www.readinga-z.com

Simms, M. (n.d.). *Sound out chapter books*. Retrieved September 7, 2009, from http://www.highnoonbooks.com

Therasimplicity. (n.d.). *Communication*. Retrieved July 2, 2009, from http://www.therasimplicity.com/

Torgesen, J., Wagner, R., & Rashotte, C. (1997). Prevention and remediation of severe reading disabilities: Keeping the end in mind. *Scientific Studies of Reading, 1*, 217–234.

VoWac Publishing Co. (n.d.). *Phonics skills for levels 1 through 4*. Retrieved September 7, 2009, from http://www.vowac.com

Wylie, R. E., & Durell, D. D. (1970). Teaching vowels through phonograms. *Elementary English, 47*(6), 787–791.

5

Across the Curriculum

Introduction

As stated in chapter 1, 80% of students with learning disabilities also have a language disability (Reed, 2005). These students may demonstrate difficulties in all academic subjects. Let us take a math story problem, for example. In order to be successful in solving these problems, students must understand the concepts and vocabulary being presented, and then they must be able to read and comprehend the problem. They must reason through how to solve the problem and then apply the math concepts to solve it. Students are expected to be successful at vocabulary and concept knowledge, decoding, encoding, reading comprehension, inferencing, and making predictions in order to solve a word problem with numbers. All subjects including language arts, social studies, science, math, and foreign languages are affected.

The use of graphic organizers can lead to greater academic success for all students. According to the National Center on Accessible Instructional Material, a graphic organizer is a visual and graphic display that shows the relationships among facts, terms, and ideas. Sometimes graphic organizers are referred to as knowledge maps, concept maps, story maps, cognitive organizers, advance organizers, semantic organizers, or concept diagrams (Hall & Strangman, 2002). According to Kim and Vaughn (2004), students with learning disabilities who used semantic organizers demonstrated significantly higher scores on researcher-developed comprehension measures than students in comparison groups. They also found that students who used visual aids outperformed those using conventional reading techniques on a reading comprehension test. Lastly, their findings indicate that the benefit of using organizers does not diminish based on grade level. Every student regardless of age or grade level can benefit from using visual strategies for academic success (Kim & Vaughn, 2004, p. 112). This chapter provides specific graphic organizers and strategies to assist students in learning across the curriculum.

Symbols and Abbreviations in Note Taking Introduction

Whether information in the classroom is presented orally or in writing, students should be encouraged in their note taking to use symbols or abbreviations whenever they can. This decreases the amount of writing and time it takes to write the notes. It also will encourage them to take notes to aid comprehension. Table 5–1 provides symbols and abbreviations that students can use.

Table 5–1. Using Symbols and Abbreviations in Note Taking

SYMBOL/ ABBREVIATION	Words/Phrases Used in Lectures	SYMBOL/ ABBREVIATION	Words/Phrases Used in Lectures
=	is equal to, is the same as	/	per
≠	is different from, unlike, is not equal to	gov. (or gvt)	government
		mbr	member
&, +	and	dept	department
>	is greater than, is more than	co.	Company
<	is less than, is smaller than	Inc.	incorporated
b/c	because, because of	mph	miles per hour
→	lead to, result in, cause to happen	st.	Street
		mfrg	manufacturing
←	result from, as a result of	mtg	meeting
↑	go up, increase, rise	mgt	management
↓	go down, decrease, drop, fall	mgr	manager
w/	with	mo/wk/yr/hr	month/week/year/hour
w/o	without	intro	introduction
w/in	within	info	information
e.g. or ex	for example, for instance	def	definition
i.e.	that is, in other words	¶	paragraph
$	money, dollar (any currency)	ch	chapter
%	percent, percentage	P or pg	page
@	at	cont	continued
# (or no.)	number	WW	World War

Note. From *Academic Skills—Standard Symbols & Abbreviations in Note-taking*, by C. Bauer-Ramazani, n.d. Retrieved February 18, 2009, from http://academics.smcvt.edu/cbauer-ramazani/IEP/acad_skills/symbols_abbrev.htm

Vocabulary Introduction

The ability to understand and accurately retrieve new vocabulary is essential for academic proficiency. In order to store and retrieve vocabulary accurately, students need to do more than memorize the words necessary for a class test. They need to understand the word in the context of the subject matter. Students need to understand multiple meanings of a word and move the vocabulary to long-term memory so that the words can be retrieved easily for use at a later time for conversation, spelling, writing, or reading. This section provides strategies to assist with learning vocabulary in order to increase storage and retrieval strength.

Vocabulary Goals

Examples of Goals

The student will increase:

1. receptive vocabulary skills including multiple meanings of words
2. receptive vocabulary skills including specific category information (this would include categories of Science, Social Studies, etc.)
3. short-term recall of newly learned vocabulary
4. long-term recall of previously learned vocabulary
5. the ability to retrieve vocabulary accurately

Vocabulary Strategies

Strategy 1: Here's How to Link Vocabulary Words With Meaning Using a Three-Dimensional Representation

The student should attempt to link new vocabulary words with a picture or idea that represents the meaning. This provides a visual strategy that the student could use if there is difficulty recalling the definition. The student may benefit from using modeling clay to make a three-dimensional representation of the vocabulary word in order to assist with recall. A picture representing the three-dimensional item can then be drawn on note cards to assist with recall while studying (Davis, 1994). The student should get to the point where he or she can visualize what would be made out of clay without actually making the item.

Strategy 2: Here's How to Create Note Cards

Using note cards provides a strategy that includes the vocabulary word, the definition, and a place to put a picture or cues to increase storage and retrieval strength. Note cards provide a study strategy, such as to study for a current test or to accumulate the vocabulary cards for unit tests or semester examinations.

Following are steps to create a note card.

Step 1: Place the note card vertically in front of the student.

Step 2: Fold the note card in half by gripping the card top edge and folding toward the student.

Step 3: Write the word on the front outside of the folded card. Write a number representing that word in the top right corner.

Step 4: Open the card and place the definition on the inside bottom of the opened card. Turn the card over and write the number that corresponds to the vocabulary word on the back of the definition section. This will permit the card to be torn in half in order to use it for matching while studying for a test. If it is a test in a vocabulary class, the word meanings should represent all of the multiple meanings of that word. If the vocabulary is subject specific, the student should concentrate on the meaning that is pertinent for that subject matter. This may be a different meaning than what the student already knows.

Step 5: Use the inside top half of the opened card to draw a picture (which may represent the three-dimensional item as listed in step 1) to assist with the semantic meaning of the word.

Step 6: If the student is experiencing word-finding difficulties, add strategies for retrieval strength (how reliably, consistently, and efficiently an item can be accessed from memory) on the inside top half of the opened card. This may include the target word, division of the word into syllables, a same-sound cue, repeating the target word, and using the word in context (German, 2007).

In the Word-Finding Intervention Program 2, German (2005) describes in detail the intervention that should be used based on the error pattern. Dr. German provides the following three error patterns for word finding.

- Error Pattern I: Lemma Related Semantic Error (Slip of the Tongue). The student with Error Pattern I is asked to rehearse his or her answer strategically before speaking. The picture used for word meaning should assist with this type of error. It will provide a visual image that the student can use to rehearse the vocabulary word before needing to use it.

- Error Pattern II: Word Form Block Error (Tip of the Tongue): Use a familiar word (a word that is usually associated with the target word (baa, baa, black sheep for black) or a same-sound word, which would be a phonological "neighbor" (related in sound, not word meaning) of the word (e.g., cell for celery).

- Error Pattern III: Word Form Phonological Error (Twist of the Tongue): Retrieves part of the word (abolism for metabolism). A three-pronged approach including a metalinguistic reinforcement, same-sound cues, and rehearsal of the single word and in context will aid in retrieval for an Error III pattern.

> **Metalinguistic:** Language meaning is greater than the words that are used. The ability to reflect consciously on the nature and properties of language (referents, multiple meaning of words, puns, riddles, humor, etc.).

Vocabulary Card Example

Table 5–2 shows an example of a vocabulary card. These cards can be used to study for a test. If the student has difficulty recalling the definition of a word, the definition can be covered. To assist with the meaning and recall of the word the student can look at the definition and retrieval cues or picture. The student can then visualize these pictures during the test to assist with word meaning and retrieval.

Strategy 3: Here's How to Use Microsoft Word® Labels to Make Vocabulary Cards

Using Microsoft Word labels offers the following benefits:

1. They decrease the need for handwriting and ensure legibility.
2. Original work is saved on the computer in case the actual cards are misplaced.

Table 5–3 shows the steps necessary for making note cards with labels in Microsoft Word 97-2003, 2007, and 2010.

The vocabulary words can be printed on labels to attach to 4 × 6 index cards in order to follow the previous strategy, or they can be printed on cardstock and folded for practice as noted in Table 5–4.

Table 5–2. Vocabulary Card Example

Outside top: 1 Number in the right upper corner that corresponds to the number on the vocabulary word		**Inside top:** Use this space to draw a picture that represents the meaning of the word. This space also can be used for word-finding strategies.
Outside bottom: 1 Vocabulary word Example: *saw*		**Inside bottom:** Definitions of the word. All definitions to multimeaning words should be written. Example: 1. A tool used for cutting 2. Past tense of *to see*

Table 5–3. Making Microsoft Labels

Word 97-2003	Word 2007	Word 2010
• Open a New Document. • Click Tools. • Click Letters/Mailings. • Click Envelopes and Labels. • Click Options. ◦ Choose the label that you are using. • Click Add Label. • Click OK. • Click New Document.	• Start Word. • On the Mailings tab, click Labels. • Leave the address box blank. • Click Options. • Click OK. • Click the type of printer that you are using to print labels. • Click the arrow next to the Label vendors' list; choose the label. • Under Print, click Full page of the same label. • Click New Document.	• Start Word. • On the Mailings tab, click Labels. • Leave the address box blank. • Click Options. • Click OK. • Click the type of printer that you are using to print labels. • Click the arrow next to the Label vendors' list; choose the label. • Under Print, click Full page of the same label. • Click New Document.

Table 5–4. Using Labels: An Example

Vocabulary Word # 1 The student should put the vocabulary word here.	**Definition for Vocabulary Word #1** The definition should go in this space so that it can be folded if not using labels.

Strategy 4: Here's How to Create Note Cards Using Greeting Card Software

Greeting card software also can be used to create note cards. The student chooses a format for a bifold card and then follows the steps listed in strategy 2. The format for making note cards and greeting cards is the same.

Strategy 5: Here's How to Learn Vocabulary Presented in a Vocabulary Class

When the curriculum includes a vocabulary class and a vocabulary building book, the following sequence should be followed in order to obtain greater understanding of the vocabulary words:

- During vocabulary unit assignments, the student should be encouraged to read the paragraph first, if presented, and then attempt to find out what the words mean by the context of the sentences and the paragraph. This provides the student with an understanding of the words in context in order to understand their meanings more completely.

- Vocabulary words should be written on note cards as suggested in strategy 2. The cards should include all meanings of the words (noun, verb, adjective, adverb, and preposition).

- Other assignments for the section are completed after the paragraph is read for meaning in context and the note cards are completed. The student should be encouraged to complete these after studying the cards. If the student can complete these assignments without looking at the words, it shows that he or she understands the words. This should assist with recall and decreased study time for testing.

In conclusion, the ability to understand vocabulary leads to the student having a more extensive vocabulary for talking, reading, and writing. This will, in turn, lead to a broader knowledge base, which will be beneficial for academic performance and test-taking skills.

Information Presented Orally Introduction

Students with language and learning disorders may have difficulty either understanding the information that is being presented orally or holding the information in short-term auditory memory long enough to follow the classroom instruction or to take notes on a classroom lecture.

Spoken Directions and Lecture Information Goals

Examples of Goals

The student will increase:

1. understanding of oral directions
2. the ability follow auditory directions
3. the ability to identify key content from auditory information
4. understanding of lecture-length information

Spoken Directions and Lecture Information Strategies

Strategy 1: Here's How to Follow Oral Directions

Often, oral directions provided are too long for many students to hold into short-term auditory memory; therefore, students should write down key words while the teacher is giving the directions. Students should be encouraged to use abbreviations or symbols.

> Teacher states, "Get your math book out of your desk, and turn to page 65. Please complete the odd number questions for questions 1–25. When you are finished, turn in your paper and finish the story that we started this morning."
>
> Student writes: math bk, pg 65, odd? 1–25, turn in, finish Turtle story.

In addition, the teacher should be encouraged to write the abbreviated version on the board so that the students can refer to the board to make sure the directions are correct.

Strategy 2: Here's How to Follow Lecture Information

- The student should preview what will be provided in the lecture. This can be accomplished by reading the sections in the textbook that will be presented or by reviewing the teacher's handouts, presentation material, or outline.

- The student should be encouraged to use Cornell Notes to take notes on lecture information. If the student has preread the information, the speech-language pathologist's or teacher's additional information should be written in the right column, so that all notes on a particular topic are together.

- If the student has not preread the information, notes should be placed in the left column during therapy or classroom lecture. When the student rereads the text, additional notes can be included in this column.

- Key points, questions, diagrams, and so on can be added to the right column as needed.

If the teacher has access to a Smart Board or PowerPoint or other visual software, the visual input will assist the student in obtaining all of the information. It also is beneficial for the student to have copies of any PowerPoint or other information the evening before the class so that he or she has the opportunity to become familiar (prelearn) before hearing it again in the classroom. If a Smart Board is used, the teacher is encouraged to print the information for the student. If the student has access to a laptop, a Cornell Notes template, Inspiration Software, or other note-taking software could be used.

In conclusion, students must develop strategies for following oral directions as well as following lecture-based material. Prereading, taking notes, and understanding the information that is presented is crucial for following a lecture in the classroom.

Following Written Directions Introduction

Students must be able to follow multistep oral directions for success in the classroom. In turn, they need to do the same with written directions. They often skip the written directions completely because they believe that they know what the directions say. Points often are missed because students do not read the directions. Underlining or highlighting key words will force students to read the directions and understand all of the steps by reviewing the key words. They can then go back after following the directions to make sure they have completed each step. Following consistent strategies for written directions will increase comprehension of the directions, thus, performance.

Following Written Directions Goals

Examples of Goals

The student will:

1. demonstrate understanding of key vocabulary while following written directions
2. increase reading comprehension for written directions
3. increase the ability to identify key high-content words while reading directions
4. follow the steps in the next section to increase understanding of written directions

Following Written Directions Strategies

Strategy 1: Here's How to Identify the Key Words

The student should be able to identify and understand key words in the direction to be able to follow it accurately. These include *list, explain, describe, compare/contrast, define, state briefly,* and *discuss.*

- *List:* Generate short answers that fit into the category of the question.
- *Describe/Explain:* Use facts and explanations in the order of how an event or action may occur.
- *Compare/Contrast:* Tell how the subjects listed in the question are the same (compare) and how they are different (contrast).
- *Define:* Provide the meaning (definition) of the word.
- *State briefly:* Provide the main idea and three supporting details.
- *Discuss:* Provide the main idea and at least three supporting details, including facts and providing explanations greater than what is expected in a brief statement.

Strategy 2: Here's How to Follow Written Directions

Now that the student can identify the important key words, it will assist in better understanding what a written direction is asking.

The student should use the following strategies for following written directions:

1. Read the direction.

2. Underline or highlight key words.

3. Follow the direction.

4. Recheck each section of the direction for accuracy.

5. Place a check mark above each part of the direction in order to assess completion of every part of it.

Following Written Directions Example

Step 1: Read the direction.
Read each sentence below. Circle the subject and underline the verb. Then write a prepositional phrase on the line to complete the sentence.

Step 2: Reread and underline or highlight key words.
Read each sentence below. Circle the subject and underline the verb. Then write a prepositional phrase on the line to complete the sentence.
or
Read each sentence below. Circle the subject and underline the verb. Then write a prepositional phrase on the line to complete the sentence.

Step 3: Follow the direction.

Step 4: Read the underlined or highlighted words. If that part of the direction has been completed, place a check mark over the completed part.

✓   ✓   ✓

Read each sentence below. Circle the subject and underline the verb. Then write a prepositional phrase on the line to complete the sentence.

In a classroom setting, teachers should be encouraged to use the directions that are written in the materials they are using or to provide the changed directions in writing. It is difficult for the student with language difficulties to get the auditory message correct or understand how to change the directions if the auditory information given is different than what is written. It also does not provide a method to check to make sure the directions were followed correctly. If the directions are altered, the teacher is encouraged to write the new direction on the board. The student should then draw a single line through the old directions then copy the new directions on the page to be completed. The teacher is encouraged to check the student's written directions for accuracy. If the changed directions are for a homework assignment, the teacher is encouraged to post the changes online through e-mail or the school's online communication system.

Strategy 3: Here's How to Follow Written Information for Math Word Problems

Solving a math word problem begins with being able to follow written directions. The second step involves understanding what question is being asked in the problem then identifying a starting point. The following steps offer an organized way to better understand and complete math word problems.

Step 1: Read the problem carefully.

Step 2: Read the problem again.
    a. Underline important words.
    b. The sentence that begins with "What" tells you what you need to solve.

Step 3: Associate numbers with important information.
    For example: A piece of property valued at $55,000 (property value = 55,000)

Step 4: Look for key words (Table 5–5).

Step 5: Identify a starting point.

Step 6: Solve the problem.

Step 7: Reread to make sure you answered the question that is being asked.

Math Story Problem Example

In 2006, Margo's first-grade class planted five trees in the front of the elementary school. Margo's class graduates in 2017. How old will the trees be when the class graduates?

Step 1: Read the problem carefully.

Step 2: Read the problem again.
    a. Underline important words.
    b. The sentence that begins with "What or How" tells you what you need to solve.

Table 5–5. Converting Words to Math Terms

English	Math
"to be" is, was, were, are	equals
amounts to, total	equals
of, times	multiplication
less than, decreased by, reduced by, fewer than	subtraction
by, total, in all, together with, combined with, more than	add

In <u>2006</u>, Margo's <u>first-grade</u> class planted five <u>trees</u> in the front of the elementary school. Margo's class <u>graduates in 2017</u>. <u>How old will</u> the <u>trees</u> be <u>when</u> the class <u>graduates?</u>

Step 3: Associate numbers with important information.

> 2006 = first grade
>
> 2017 = graduation

Step 4: Look for key words.
First grade planted trees in 2006. Graduates in 2017. How old will the trees be?

Step 5: Identify a starting point.
Need to find out how many years between 2006 and 2017.

Step 6: Solve the problem.

$$\begin{array}{r} 2017 \\ -2006 \\ \hline 11 \end{array}$$

Step 7: Reread to make sure you answered the question that is being asked.
The trees will be 11 years old.

In conclusion, many students miss points on assignments not because they do not know the answer but because they complete the assignment or question without reading the directions. This often happens because the student thinks that the question is similar to one already completed, so it must have the same directions. The assignment or question may be slightly or completely different whereby not reading the directions leads to incorrect or partial answers.

Reading Comprehension Introduction

Listening comprehension skills are strongly related to reading comprehension skills (Diakidoy, Styllianou, Karefillidou, & Papageorgiou, 2005; Hagtvet, 2003; Nation & Snowling, 2004). Therefore, students with difficulty with listening comprehension are at risk for reading comprehension difficulties.

The ability to understand information presented in written format begins at a very young age with beginning reading. Beginning books typically have one or two sentences per page then gradually increase in number of words in the sentence and then number of words on a page. These are vital steps in order for the student to comprehend the words on the page with increasing length and complexity. The following section provides strategies for reading comprehension. For comprehension of any length of information, the student should use any pictures, charts, or graphs that may be on the page to best understand the information being presented. After scanning across the page in order to have a general idea of the information, the next step is to read the written information.

Reading Comprehension for Paragraph-Length Information Goals

Examples of Goals

The student will increase the ability to:

1. comprehend paragraph-length information
2. choose high-content information from a paragraph
3. identify the main idea
4. provide three relevant details to support the main idea

Paragraph-Length Material Strategies

Strategy 1: Here's How to Scan and Read Paragraph-Length Information

The student should be encouraged to scan all of the information that is presented on the page before beginning to read. This provides an overview of the information. It also provides the student the opportunity to begin finding out what is already known about the material. The following steps should be followed for each paragraph:

1. Visually scan information and any pictures or other information provided.
2. Read.
3. Reread/underline important information.
4. Identify the main idea.
5. Provide three details from the story that support the main idea.

Paragraph-Length Information Example

1. Scan the page for information.
2. Read the story.

> One sunny Saturday morning, Johnny and his family went to the neighborhood park. The first thing Johnny did was to run to the slides. He played on the slides for 10 minutes. After he was finished swinging, he saw his friend, Susie, playing on the monkey bars. They played together until it was time to eat the picnic lunch that Johnny's parents packed. Johnny asked if Susie could eat lunch with them. Both Johnny's and Susie's parents said that it was all right for Susie to eat with Johnny's family. When lunch was finished, the student played in the sandbox for a few minutes until it was time to go home. Johnny had a wonderful day at the park.

3. Reread the story and underline important information.

One <u>sunny Saturday morning</u>, <u>Johnny and his family</u> went to the <u>neighborhood park</u>. The first thing <u>Johnny</u> did was to run to the <u>slides</u>. He played on the <u>slides for 10 minutes</u>. <u>After</u> he was <u>finished sliding</u>, he <u>saw</u> his friend, <u>Susie</u>, playing <u>on</u> the <u>monkey bars</u>. They <u>played together until</u> it was time to eat the picnic <u>lunch that Johnny's parents packed</u>. Johnny asked <u>if Susie could eat lunch with them</u>. Both Johnny's and Susie's parents said that <u>it was all right for Susie to eat</u> with Johnny's family. When <u>lunch was finished</u>, the student <u>played in the sandbox</u> for a few minutes <u>until</u> it was <u>time to go</u> home. Johnny had a wonderful day at the park.

4. Main idea: Johnny had a great day at the park.

5. Three details to support the main idea:
   a. Played on the slide, monkey bars, and sandbox
   b. Played with his friend Susie
   c. Had a picnic lunch

Strategy 2: Here is How to Use Graphic Organizers

Another strategy to assist in the organization of information for greater comprehension is a graphic organizer. The information can be placed into the organizer so that it is easier to ascertain what the main idea is and the details that support it. Graphic organizers assist the student with separating the main idea from the supporting details to increase comprehension of the presented information.

A web, as shown in Figure 5–1 from Microsoft Word, provides a visual representation of information in a paragraph. It assists with finding the main idea of the paragraph and the details that support the main idea, thus increasing comprehension of the material.

Microsoft Word 97-2003 has concept maps, such as webs for visual support, under the drawing toolbar. Go to the drawing toolbar. Double-click on the cycle diagram icon to pull up Options for visual supports. These include an organizational chart, a Venn diagram, cycle diagram, web, pyramid, and a target diagram. In Windows 2007 and 2010, go to Insert. Click on SmartArt. Options for visual support will be displayed.

Software programs such as Inspiration Software and ReadWriteThink offer concept mapping options as well. Inspiration Software webs feature the ability to add pictures and other graphics to support information. This program then allows the student to click on the outline icon, which will move the information that was webbed to an outline format. This assists in the student's organization as well as provides a means to move to an outline format quickly if required by the teacher (Inspiration Software, Inc., n.d.). ReadWriteThink (n.d.) offers several graphic organizers that can be printed but does not have a Save option to be able to add information once the window for the Web site is closed.

In conclusion, once the student is able to develop strategies for comprehension of paragraph-length information, chapter length or greater will follow the same format because even though there is a greater amount of information, it is still divided into paragraph length.

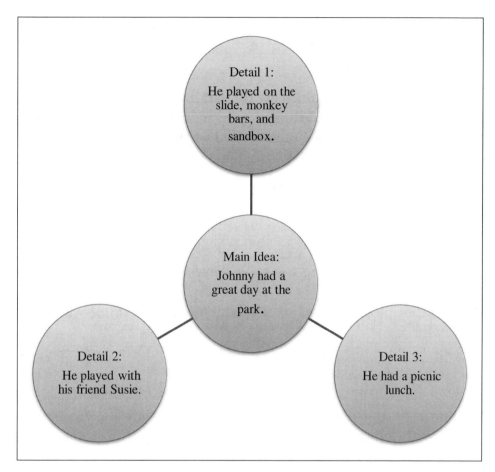

Figure 5–1. Using a Concept Map: Web.

Reading Comprehension for Subject-Based Information Goals

Examples of Goals

The student will increase reading comprehension for:

1. paragraph-length information
2. chapter-length information
3. book-length information

Subject-Based Information Strategies

Strategy 1: Here's How to Use KWL

During Social Studies, Science, and any other areas that require a significant amount of reading, assist the student in following the Know, What, Learn (KWL) format:

1. Know: What I know
2. What: What I want to know
3. Learn: What I learned

The student will be more successful if new content area is built upon what the student already knows. For example, if the student went on a family vacation to Mount Rushmore, pictures of Mount Rushmore should be used when discussing the area, type of rock, geographical location, and so on.

Strategy 2: Here's How to Use SQ3R

SQ3R is an acronym that stands for Scan, Questions, Read, Recite, and Review. The following provides specific information for each step of SQ3R.

Step 1: Scan: Survey the chapter including chapter and section titles, pictures, graphs, charts, and captions.
   a. Read the title of the chapter: This will provide the framework of the chapter content.
   b. Read the title of the lesson: This will provide information about the specific lesson within the chapter.
   c. Read the subsection title: This will provide the framework for the subsection.

Step 2: Question: The student should reflect on what is already known about the chapter then turn the chapter and section titles into a question to be answered after reading that section or the entire chapter (for the chapter title question).

Step 3: Read: The student should try answering the questions posed in step 2 while reading.

Step 4: Recite: State the answers to the section question. The student should reread the section before moving to the next one if unable to answer questions about the section. At this point, the student should take notes regarding the new learning. Microsoft labels or 4 × 6 note cards, as described in this chapter for vocabulary, also can be used for note taking (Table 5–6).

Step 5: Review: The student should be encouraged to look at notes each day in order to completely grasp and remember the information.

In summary, SQ3R provides another strategy to assist with comprehension of subject-based information in order to understand and retain newly learned information.

Strategy 3: Here's How to Use Cornell Notes

A very popular method of note taking for middle school, high school, and college students is the Cornell method created by Walter Pauk in the 1950s. This strategy can be used while prereading an assignment or while taking notes in class.

Notes column (right): In keeping with the idea that many students with language-based learning disabilities should prelearn information before class, it is recommended that they take notes using this column while they are reading the information before it

Table 5–6. Using Microsoft Labels for Note Taking

Front of the Card	Back of the Card (Summary)
(Section title) Immigration and Citizenship	• Immigration has shaped the history and people of the United States. • The United States continues to have the most open immigration laws in the world. *This section can be used to add comments by the teacher*

is presented in therapy or class. If the student has not preread the information, he or she writes information from the lecture on the right side, keeping the sentences very brief. The student should use bulleted lists for easy skimming and as many abbreviations or symbols as possible (without sacrificing readability and understanding when reviewing the notes.). Only one subsection or topic should be written on each sheet of paper. This will permit more information about the topic to be added. It also will keep all of the notes regarding one topic in one place, thus assisting with organization.

Cues column (left): After taking notes (either from prereading and adding the teacher's notes to the right or after taking lecture notes) the student can use this section to write the main idea, add diagrams or charts, write vocabulary words, or write questions that need clarification in the left column that help connect ideas listed in the notes section. When studying, the student should look at the cues in this column to help recall the facts (details that support the main idea) in notes.

Summary area (bottom): The summary section at the bottom is used to summarize all of the information into one or two sentences.

Cornell Notes Example

Table 5–7 shows an example of Cornell Notes.

Strategy 4: Here's How to Study and Review Using Cornell-Formatted Notes

The student may need assistance regarding how and when to take Cornell Notes. A discussion should also occur regarding how these notes will assist the student when listening to lecture information in class as well as utilizing the notes to study for upcoming tests. The following steps are encouraged.

1. Preread before class and take notes in the right column. If the student does not preread (although strongly recommended for retention), he or she should take classroom notes in the right column.

Table 5–7. Example of Cornell Notes*

Name: _____

Class: _____

Cues	Notes
This section is written after the right side is completed.	These are the notes that the student should take while prereading to prepare for the next class in a subject. If the student does not preread, this is where classroom notes are taken.
✓ Main Ideas ✓ Diagrams/Graphs ✓ Vocabulary ✓ ? for clarification	The student should use a separate page for each subsection in the textbook. This will allow room to add the teacher's information or further information while reading.
◄──────► 2½ inches	◄──────────────► 6 inches

Summary

While studying, the student should write one or two sentence summary.   2 inches

*Cornell Notes were developed by Walter Pauk in the 1950s. He was a professor at Cornell University in the Department of Developmental Education and Study Skills (Pauk, 2007).

2. Use single sheets for each subsection.

3. While reviewing the notes, write down the main ideas, diagrams, vocabulary, questions for clarification, and so on in the left column.

4. Write a one or two-sentence summary at the bottom.

5. When the time comes to study for an exam, the student should do the following:
    a. Read through the Cornell Notes.
    b. Quiz oneself. Cover up the right side and use the cues on the left to assist with memory and retrieve details.
    c. Uncover the right side to check for retrieval of facts.

Using the Cornell Method and Underlining Key Words Example

Table 5–8 provides an example of how the Cornell method is used to write notes.

Clara Barton

Born on December 25, 1821, in Oxford, Massachusetts, the youngest of 5 children in a middle-class family, Barton was educated at home, and at fifteen started teaching school. Her most notable antebellum achievement was the establishment of a free public school in Bordentown, N.J. Though she is remembered as the founder of the American Red Cross, her only prewar medical experience came when for two years she nursed an invalid brother.

Table 5–8. Using Cornell Notes

Name: _____

Class: Social Studies: Clara Barton

Main Ideas	Notes on Clara Barton

✓ Clara Barton led a life of service as
  ○ Educator
  ○ Caregiver
 	
Definition:
Middle class: The socioeconomic class between the working class and the upper class. Professionals and skilled laborers are usually said to be in this class.
 	
Question:
Did Clara's upbringing lead her to help others?
	✓ Born: 12/25/1821 in Oxford, MA
	✓ Youngest of 5
	✓ Took care of sick brother
	✓ Educated at home
	✓ Began teaching @ 15
	✓ Opened a free public school in Bordentown, NJ
	✓ Helped soldiers during Civil War
	✓ Organized med. supplies from donations
	✓ Cared for soldiers in Fredericksburg, VA
	✓ Founded the Am. Red Cross in 1881
	✓ Head of Red Cross until 1904
	✓ Died Apr. 12, 1912

Summary

Clara Barton was a teacher and wanted all students to have an education. She also saw a need for medical supplies on the battle field during the Civil War. Clara Barton founded the first public education as well as the Am. Red Cross

In 1861, Barton was living in Washington, D.C., working at the U.S. Patent Office. When the 6th Massachusetts Regiment arrived in the city after the Baltimore Riots, she organized a relief program for the soldiers, beginning a lifetime of philanthropy. When Barton learned that many of the wounded from First Bull Run had suffered, not from want of attention but from need of medical supplies, she advertised for donations in the Worcester, Mass., *Spy* and began an independent organization to distribute goods. The relief operation was successful, and the following year U.S. Surgeon General William A. Hammond granted her a general pass to travel with army ambulances "for the purpose of distributing comforts for the sick and wounded, and nursing them."

For 3 years she followed army operations throughout the Virginia theater and in the Charleston, S.C., area. Her work in Fredericksburg, Va., hospitals, caring for the casualties from the Battle of the Wilderness, and nursing work at Bermuda Hundred attracted national notice. At this time she formed her only formal Civil War connection with any organization when she served as superintendent of nurses in Maj. Gen. Benjamin F. Butlers command.

She also expanded her concept of soldier aid, traveling to Camp Parole, Md., to organize a program for locating men listed as missing in action. Through interviews with Federals returning from Southern prisons, she was often able to determine the status of some of the missing and notify families.

By the end of the war Barton had performed most of the services that would later be associated with the <u>American Red Cross</u>, which she <u>founded in 1881</u>. In <u>1904 she resigned</u> as head of that organization, retiring to her home at Glen Echo, outside Washington, D.C., where she <u>died 12 Apr. 1912.</u> (Weeks, n.d.)

In conclusion, the student can learn strategies that can be used across the curriculum regardless of the subject matter. Some students will need additional support to find out how these strategies can be used for all course material.

Reading Comprehension for Literature Goals

Example of Goals

The student will increase comprehension of books containing chapter length material with increasing complexity to include:

1. Leveled readers in order to achieve appropriate reading level
2. Chapter books with two to three pages per chapter
3. Chapter books with three to eight pages per chapter
4. Chapter books with more than eight pages per chapter

Reading Comprehension for Literature Strategies

Strategy 1: Here's How to Use a Book Report Format for Documentation

A book report format will encourage the student to be sure that the information that he or she is reading is understood before moving on to the next chapter. The student should use the following steps while preparing to and reading a book:

1. Read the summary presented on the back of the book (or the paper cover).
2. Use a book report format to write information gained from the book summary (Form 5–1). This will typically include:
   a. Plot (the main idea or what the story is about)
      i. It is the sequence of events in a story or play—what happens first, second, third, and ongoing. The short story usually has one plot so it can be read in one sitting.
   b. Main character or characters
      i. The person
      ii. The characteristics of a person (what the character is like)
         a) his or her physical appearance
         b) what he or she says or thinks
         c) what he or she does or does not do
         d) how others react or view this character

■ FORM 5–1. Using a Book Report Format

Book Report

Name: _____   Date: _____

Book Title: _____   Illustrator: _____

Author: _____   Publisher: _____

Due Dates of Assignments:

Assignment:	Due Date:

Plot (*Main idea of the story*)

```



```

Setting (*Describe the time, location, climate, and mood of the story*)

```



```

Main characters (*Describe the main character and his/her characteristics (physical appearance, what he or she does, etc.)*

```



```

continues

continued

Conflict or central problem (*Describe the main problem or conflict the characters have to solve*)

Main idea and three details from each chapter

Resolution of the conflict (*At what point was the conflict resolved? How was it resolved?*)

Conclusion (*Tell how the book ended*)

Your thoughts on this book (*Tell whether you liked or disliked the book and give three reasons for your opinion*)

      c. Setting (the time and location [where] in which a story takes place)
          i. Place: Geographical location. Where is the action of the story taking place?
          ii. Time: When is the story taking place? (Historical period, time of day, year, etc)
          iii. Weather conditions: Is it rainy, sunny, stormy, . . . ?
          iv. Mood: What feeling is created at the beginning of the story? Is it bright and cheerful or dark and frightening?
      d. Conflict or central problem (the problem that the main character must solve)

3. Use the information entered into the book report format to refer to while reading and also to add further information learned while reading.

4. Write the main idea and at least three supporting details about the chapter before reading the next one. If the student is unable to recall details, the chapter should be skimmed or reread before moving forward.

5. Additional characters/characteristics as well as additional information learned about the characters should be included as the information is presented.

6. When the student reaches the point of the climax (how the conflict is resolved) of the story, he or she should complete that section.

7. After completing the story, the student completes the section regarding how the story ended.

8. Finally, the student should reflect on the story and complete the section regarding whether the book was liked or disliked. This requires the student to use critical thinking in order to provide details of why the story or book was liked or disliked. This is crucial in order to build a desire to read more books of a particular genre or to try books of a different genre if the student did not like the book.

Many books are now available on CD or MP3 so that students can listen to a story. They should be encouraged to follow along in the book. This will increase identification of sight words, vocabulary skills, and, thus, accuracy. Most new textbooks are available on audio as well. The texts also typically have workbooks and leveled supplemental reading material to support the textbook.

In conclusion, a book report format will assist the student with gathering information before beginning to read the book by reviewing the summary. This will provide information regarding the characters, plot, and setting. In addition, it will provide the student with basic information to begin making predictions regarding the story content. The student then documents the key points of each chapter. If the chapters have titles, the student can then make the chapter title into a question to make sure that he or she understands the main idea and supporting details before moving on to the next chapter.

Reading Comprehension and Critical Thinking Goals

Examples of Goals

The student will increase:

1. comprehension of the reading material in order to infer information from what is read
2. the ability to make predictions from read material

Reading Comprehension and Critical Thinking Strategies

Strategy 1: Here's How to Use Critical Thinking

The student should be encouraged to attempt the critical thinking tasks during every therapy session. He or she also should be encouraged to complete these tasks in Science and Social Studies chapter reviews even if not assigned. This will assist in a deeper understanding of the material. For compare and contrast questions, the student should make a chart. The speech-language pathologist or educator may need to explain the following concepts before the assignment begins: compare = how are they the same; contrast = how are they different (Table 5–9).

Compare and Contrast Example

Table 5–10 provides an example of an exercise comparing and contrasting two seasons.

A T chart also can be used if the student needs to compare or contrast two subjects. Each subject can be written on the horizontal line with the vertical line separating the two areas.

A Venn diagram can be used to compare and contrast topics (Figure 5–2). The Venn diagram provides a visual strategy to easily organize how topics are the same and how they are different. The outer section of each circle represents the information that is unique to one of the topics. Where the circles overlap represents the information that the topics have in common.

Table 5–9. T Chart Compare/Contrast

Compare	Contrast
How the topics are the same (what they have in common)	How the topics are different (what is not the same about the topics)

Table 5–10. Compare and Contrast the Seasons of Winter and Spring Example

Compare (how are they the same)	Contrast (how are they different)
• They are both seasons. • In some areas of the world, the climate is the same regardless of season. • They occur at the same time each calendar year. • Global warming has made the seasons warmer.	• They occur at different times of the calendar year. • Weather patterns are different. • Types of weather depend on geographical location.

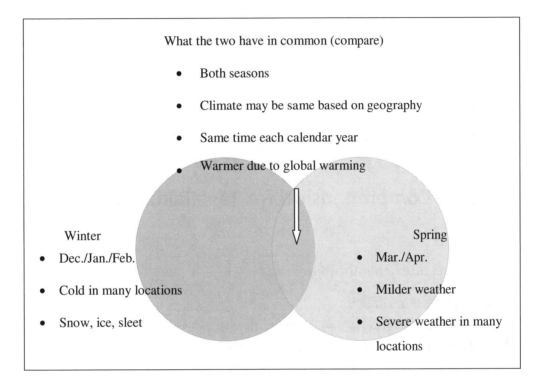

Figure 5–2. Venn Diagrams: Comparing Two Subjects.

A three-circle Venn diagram works well for areas of Science or Social Studies where three similar subjects are compared and contrasted; for example: comparing and contrasting three wars, historical figures, types of rocks, periods, and others. The section where two topics overlap would represent what those two topics have in common. The middle section where all circles overlap represents what all of the topics have in common (Figure 5–3).

In conclusion, students must be able to use critical thinking for learning. This allows them to learn new information and know how it applies to what is already known. Critical thinking also provides a way to study for tests. It allows the student to develop ways to retrieve information during testing if the information can be related to the gestalt of the general information.

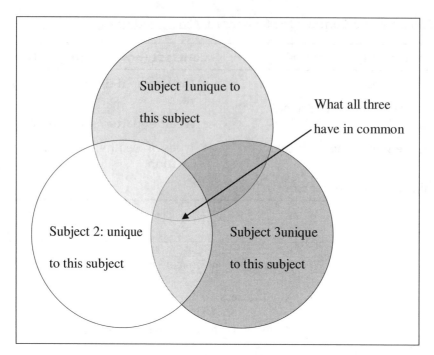

Figure 5–3. Venn Diagram: Comparing Three Subjects.

Reading Comprehension for Test-Taking Strategies

Examples of Goals

The student will increase generalization of:

1. following written directions
2. information read in order to reiterate it with details and provide critical thinking regarding the material
3. learned main ideas and supporting details

Reading Comprehension for Test-Taking Strategies

Strategy 1: Here's How to Use a Word Bank

Students should be encouraged to group words together in the word bank in order to limit correct answers to a question. For example, they should use an abbreviation to place by each word in order to put it in a category (p = person, pl = place, t = thing, d = date, e = event).

Grouping Words During a Test Example

When answering a question from the word bank, students can limit choices for the correct answer by understanding if the question is asking for a person, place, thing, date, or event (Table 5–11).

Table 5–11. Grouping Words During Testing

December 25, 1821	d	Oxford, MA	pl	Free public education	t
Clara Barton	p	Civil War	e	Worcester, MA	pl
Washington, DC	pl	Benjamin Butler	p	American Red Cross	t
1861	d	Charleston, SC	pl	Relief operation	t
William Hammond	p	Camp Parole, MD	pl	Battle of Wilderness	e
First Bull Run	e	April 12, 1912	d		

Strategy 2: Here's How to Follow Directions or Paragraph-Length Information on a Test

The student should underline or highlight key words for what is required on each portion of the test as well as underline important words in each test question, just as demonstrated in the section Following Written Directions. First and foremost, this requires that the student read the direction instead of assuming understanding of the question being asked. Second, it assists in picking up on key words, such as *not*, in a direction. It also provides an avenue to check answers for completion. The student should pay particular attention to the key words (*list, explain, describe, compare/contrast, define, state briefly, discuss*) that were provided in the section Following Written Directions.

Strategy 3: Here's How to Answer Questions That Require Writing a Sentence or a Paragraph

If the student has to write a short answer or essay that requires him or her to explain, describe, compare/contrast, state briefly, or discuss, using visual supports such as a Venn diagram or web is helpful to organize information as a prewriting task. This assists with organizing thoughts before beginning to write. It also assists with obtaining the main idea and supporting details (Figure 5–4).

The student also can use a compare/contrast chart such as that presented earlier to respond in a written format for a compare and contrast question on a test (Table 5–12).

In addition, a Venn diagram can be used while answering a compare and contrast question on an examination (Figure 5–5).

Strategy 4: Here's How to Answer True and False Questions

- Instruct the student to look for absolute words that usually indicate a false statement.
  - *Never, All, None, Always*
- Instruct the student to look for general words that usually indicate a true statement.
  - *Frequently, Usually, Sometimes, Generally*

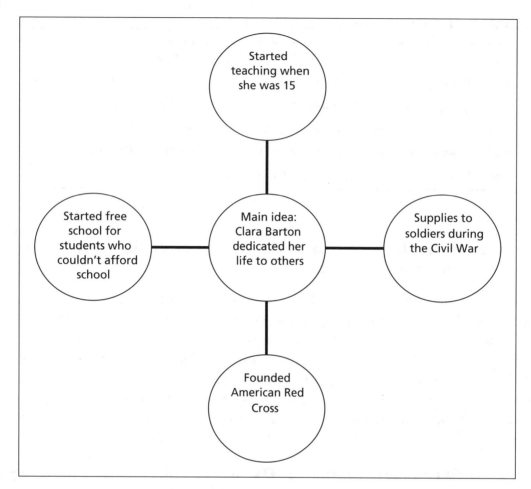

Figure 5–4. Example Using Webbing.

Table 5–12. Using Compare/Contrast Chart Example 2

Essay Question: Compare and contrast the life of Clara Barton with your favorite hero.		
	Compare	**Contrast**
Clara Barton and Dorothea Lange	No formal training Both women helped others Social conscience	Clara: teacher, organizer, Civil War, helped others due to upbringing, American Red Cross Dorothea: photographer, Great Depression, social awareness due to firsthand experience with a disability

Strategy 5: Here's How to Answer Multiple Choice Questions

- Instruct the student to look for words such as *all, none, not, never, always.*

- Instruct the student to place a single line through any statements that cannot be the answer to the question. This will reduce the number of choices to correctly answer the question.

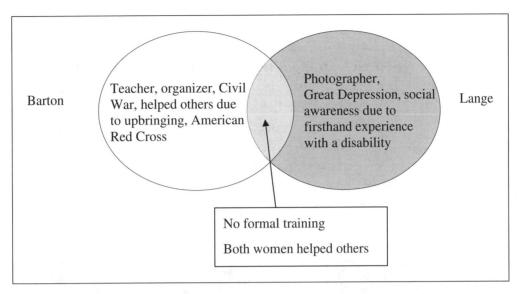

Figure 5–5. Example Using a Venn Diagram.

Strategy 6: Here's How to Skip Questions Unable to Answer

- The student should be instructed to use a sticky tab to mark any questions that were skipped. This will remind him or her to go back and answer the questions before turning in the test.

- The purpose for skipping questions are twofold:
  - Extra time is not spent trying to come up with or retrieve the answer.
  - There may be additional questions on the test provided in a different format that would provide information in order to go back and correctly answer the question.

Strategy 7: Here's How to Take Open-Book or Open-Note Tests

- Students should be encouraged to use the Cornell Notes or concept maps made while reading the chapter(s).
  - Page numbers that correspond to where the information was found in the book should be added in a different color.

- Students also should use sticky tabs with the section information or important vocabulary written on the tab so that it is easier to find the information. These tabs should be in order with the beginning chapter information being placed on the tab that will be at the top of the page. Each subsequent tab should be placed lower so it is easily read.

- Students should be encouraged to answer any questions they know without looking up the information. Additional information can be added if time allows.

In conclusion, all of the strategies that are presented in this chapter can be used during test taking to understand what is being asked as well as to organize thoughts in order to provide clear and concise answers.

Conclusion

Students with language-based learning disabilities will demonstrate difficulty across all academic areas. This is because language is involved in every academic area. The strategies presented in this chapter will provide the student with skills that can be applied across the curriculum. These strategies can be used for following oral and written directions every time a direction is presented. Graphic organizers will provide a clear and concise way to manage information. These strategies can then be applied during test taking in order to follow the directions for each section of the examination, to answer questions, and to apply critical thinking for question completion.

References

Bauer-Ramazani, C. (n.d.). *Academic skills—standard symbols & abbreviations in note-taking.* Retrieved February 18, 2009, from http://academics.smcvt.edu/cbauer-ramazani/IEP/acad_skills/symbols_abbrev.htm

Davis, R. (1994). *The gift of dyslexia.* New York, NY: Ability Workshop Press.

Diakidoy, I. A., Styllianou, P., Karefillidou, C., & Papageorgiou, P. (2005). The relationship between listening and reading comprehension of different types of tests at increasing grade levels. *Reading Psychology, 26,* 55–80.

German, D. (2005). *Word finding intervention program 2.* Austin, TX: Pro-Ed.

German, D. (2007). *Dual-focus vocabulary instruction for word finding, meanings, and retrieval strategies.* Lecture conducted from American Speech-Language-Hearing Association National Convention, Boston, MA.

Hagtvet, B. E. (2003). Listening comprehension and reading comprehension in poor decoders: Evidence for the importance of syntactic and semantic skill as well as phonological skills. *Reading and Writing: An Interdisciplinary Journal, 16,* 505–539.

Hall, T., & Strangman, N. (2002). *Graphic organizers.* Wakefield, MA: National Center on Accessing the General Curriculum. Retrieved February 13, 2011, from http://aim.cast.org/learn/historyarchive/backgroundpapers/graphic_organizers

Inspiration Software, Inc. (n.d.). Inspiration 9: 5-12 [Computer program]. Retrieved February 6, 2009, from http://www.inspiration.com

Kim, A., & Vaughn, S. (2004). Graphic organizers and their effects on the reading comprehension of students with LD: A synthesis of research. *Journal of Learning Disabilities, 37*(2), 105–118. Retrieved December 6, 2010, from http://www.asha.org

McGraw-Hill Student's Publishing. (1998). *Thinking skills grade 5.* Columbus, OH: Author.

Nation, K., & Snowling, M. J. (2004). Beyond phonological skills: Broader language skills contribute to the development of reading. *Journal of Research in Reading, 27,* 342–356.

Pauk, W. (2007). *How to study in college.* Boston, MA: Houghton Mifflin.

ReadWriteThink. (n.d.). *Student interactive story map.* Retrieved February 6, 2009, from http://www.readwritethink.org/student_mat/index.asp

Reed, V. (2005). *An introduction to children with language disorders* (3rd ed.). Boston, MA: Pearson/Allyn and Bacon.

Remedia Publications. (1998). *Test-taking strategies.* Scottsdale, AZ: Author.

Weeks, R. (n.d.). *Clara Harlowe Barton. The American Civil War.* Retrieved February 18, 2009, from http://civilwarhome.com/bartonbio

6

Expressing Oneself Through Writing

Introduction

Children with preschool speech and language disorders often are considered at risk for school-age reading, writing, and spelling difficulties (Singer, 1995). Research also reveals that children with language impairment (LI) produce written texts that have fewer words, syntax errors, and poorer organization, similar to their oral language (Bishop & Clarkson, 2003; Dockrell, Lindsay, Connelly, & Mackie, 2007; Singer & Bashir, 2004; Scott and Windsor, 2000).

Besides those with language impairments, students, overall, are demonstrating a lack of proficiency with written language. According to the National Assessment of Educational Progress (NAEP), in 2002 only 28% of 4th graders, 31% of 8th graders, and 24% of 12th graders performed at or above the proficient level of writing as defined as solid academic performance for grade level (Lutkus, Weiner, Daane, & Jin, 2003). In 2007, 165,000 students in the 8th and 12th grades throughout the nation were reassessed. The following results were obtained:

- For 8th grade, the percentage of students performing at or above the proficient level showed no significant change since 2002.

- For 12th grade, the percentage of students performing at or above the proficient level showed no significant change since 2002 (Salahu-Din, Persky, and Miller, 2008).

A written language disorder is described by Dr. Margaret Kay (2007) as a highly complex neurodevelopmental process that requires simultaneous and sequential integration of attention, multiple information sources, visual memory, motor skills, language (morphology, phonology, semantics, syntax, pragmatics, and metalinguistic skills), and higher cognition.

As stated in the preceding definition, a disorder of written language expression involves many of the areas that we see in students with a speech and/or language disorder. Written expression, or written language expression, relies on mastery of many language areas. This includes receptive and expressive vocabulary. Students must possess age-appropriate vocabulary skills in order to write about age-appropriate topics. This includes multiple word meanings, synonyms, and antonyms. They also must have adequate phonological awareness and phonics skills in order to correctly spell the words used in the written expression. In addition, students have to demonstrate age-appropriate receptive and expressive language skills for morphology, semantics, and syntax., Students need to have the ability to do the following: understand and use similes, metaphors, and idioms; follow auditory and/or written directions in order to understand the requirements of the writing assignment; and retrieve words and information quickly and accurately. Appropriate reading comprehension also is needed if they have to answer questions in writing based on a paragraph or a story. In addition to all of these areas, students must be able to organize the information that will be included in the written format.

In 1993, Judith Osgood Smith conducted a study in which 31 college students with documented learning disabilities were interviewed. The students were asked to rate themselves regarding the demands and difficulty of written requirements in college. This included the following areas:

Writing requirements
- Out of class papers/reports
- Questions based on readings
- Other (article critiques)

Aspect of Writing Difficulty
- Detecting errors/proofreading
- Grammar
- Spelling
- Writing (speed and legibility)
- Organizing thoughts
- Locating relevant information
- Typing/word processing

The area that the students rated as the most difficult was detecting errors/proof reading—71% of the students stated that they could not recognize errors, which included incorrect spelling, language structure, and grammar usage. In regard to grammar, 64.5% rated it as very or extremely difficult. This included feeling ill prepared during high school and having problems with mechanics of writing. Spelling was found extremely difficult by 54.8% of the students. This included difficulty remembering or applying spelling rules, problems with memory, and the ability to sound out words. Writing and/or legibility was rated as difficult by 51.6% of the students. They mentioned frustration with putting ideas on paper, thus increasing frustration and then decreasing legibility. There were 48.4% who reported organizing thoughts as difficult as they prepared to write. This included keeping the topic in focus, simplifying and condensing information into an organized fashion, as well as deciding which ideas went together. Strengths included typing/word processing and locating relevant information.

This information, compared to the NAEP for writing, demonstrates that ongoing written language difficulties will continue after high school if proficiency is not accomplished by the time the students graduate from high school.

Katz et al. (2007) conducted a survey of 693 school-based speech-language pathologists (SLPs) regarding their level of knowledge and attitudes toward provision of written language services. The survey found that 52% of the participants felt they did have the overall expertise to help struggling readers and writers. The greatest amount of knowledge was reported for phonological awareness (92% strongly agreed or agreed). The least amount of knowledge was reported for spelling (42% strongly agreed or agreed), expository writing skills (46% strongly agreed or agreed), and narrative writing skills (51% strongly agreed or agreed). Furthermore, SLPs reported providing written language services to only 43% of students who needed these services. There were 225 SLPs who identified students on their caseload as having written language needs, and they did not provide any services to these students in the area of written language.

Written language expression is the culmination of many expressive language areas (morphology, phonology, semantics, syntax, word finding) and auditory comprehension areas (morphology, phonology, semantics, and syntax). It also requires metalinguistic knowledge and use. This chapter discusses the components needed to have adequate written language. It concentrates on written language skills from third grade through high school. This chapter introduces some basic lessons of writing, strategies for organization of written expression for answering questions, how to use writing prompts, how to write a summary/essay, and how to develop a more in-depth paper. It also includes accommodations, compensatory strategies, and bypass strategies.

Assessment Tools Review

Several standardized tools that measure writing ability are listed in chapter 2, Diagnostics. A description of what each test measures is included as well. The tests include:

- *OWLS* Written Portion (Carrow-Woolfolk, 1996)
- The *Test of Written Language* (Hammil, Brown, & Larsen, 2009)
- The *Test of Early Written Language* (Hresko, Herron, & Peak, 2001)
- *Woodcock-Johnson II* (Woodcock, McGrew, & Mather, 2001)
- *Wechsler Individual Achievement Test III* (Wechsler, 2009)

An informal assessment of writing also can occur. The following areas should be evaluated:

- Use of vocabulary
- Use of syntax
- Spelling
- Mechanics (capitalization, punctuation, paragraph formulation)
- Grammar
- Cohesiveness (clear and logical relationships among ideas)
- Coherence (writing is logical and connected)
- Overall quality (The 5 Cs: Clear, Concise, Compelling, Consistent, and Correct)

Strategies to Improve Writing Skills Introduction

There are so many areas to consider when assisting students with written language. First, the topic for writing must be understood or generated. Second, ideas have to be generated. Third, the ideas have to be organized. Next, the main idea needs to be expressed. Details surrounding the main idea must be organized. The student needs to consider how to conclude the writing. All of this must be considered before the student begins the actual writing process. Next, there is the prewriting and writing process. This process is then followed by proofing. We can use several strategies to assist with the entire process.

Here's How to Use Strategies to Assist With Written Language

- Idea Generation
  Depending on the writing assignment, the student may need to generate lists of words or ideas that could be associated with the topic. The student can then use a numbering system in order to put like ideas together. Once the like ideas are together, a graphic organizer such as a web, T chart, or Venn diagram can be used for prewriting and organizing the ideas.

  For example, if the writing assignment asked for the student to plan a birthday party, the following ideas could be generated.

cake	Pin the Tail on the Donkey	balloons
ice cream	Relay Races	party bags
pizza	Musical Chairs	candles

  Once the ideas are generated, numbers can be assigned to represent items that go together.

1 cake	2 Pin the Tail on the Donkey	3 balloons
1 ice cream	2 Relay Races	3 party bags
1 pizza	2 Musical Chairs	3 candles

1 = food,   2 = games   3 = supplies needed

Here's How to Use Webs, Venn Diagrams, and Other Graphic Organizers

Graphic organizers are a very successful way to assist students with organizing their thoughts. A web can be used for written language of five sentences to five or more paragraphs. Chapter 5, Across the Curriculum, provides examples of using webs. First, the student organizes the main idea (middle bubble), at least three supporting details (bubbles surrounding the main idea), and an idea for a conclusion (bubble surrounding the main idea). For younger students, I ask them to write complete sentences in the bubbles. This makes it very easy to move from the prewriting of the web to the paragraph. It also helps them organize their thoughts to write the sentence. The bubble size also seems to assist them to not have run-on sentences. Once the students are proficient with writing grammatically correct sentences, it is acceptable to place key words in the bubbles. The actual sentence generation occurs during the draft.

The web can be used to write several paragraphs. Each bubble would represent the idea for a paragraph. The main idea then becomes the thesis statement when writing.

If the student is required to compare and contrast information, a Venn diagram provides an ideal visual organizer. This may need to be a preliminary step in organizing ideas. The student may then need to web this information in order to organize the information for writing.

Here Are Programs for Writing

- Step Up to Writing
  Step Up to Writing is a program that is often used in the classroom for expository writing (inform, explain, describe, or define the subject). It teaches writing strategies within the writing process (prewriting, drafting, revising, editing, final copy, proofreading, sharing) to help students organize their thinking and their writing. Each element of expository writing (thesis statement, topic sentences, transitions, examples, and conclusion) is color coded in the organization phase (Auman, 1999).

- The Writing Lab Approach to Language Instruction
  The Writing Lab Approach to Language Instruction provides computer-supported activities that focus on the five language domains—morphology, phonology, semantics, syntax, and pragmatics (Wolf Nelson, Barh, & Van Meter, 2004).

- The Story Grammar Marker
  The Story Grammar Marker uses manipulative tools and resources that help students in Grades 2 through 6 develop reading, writing, and speaking skills (Moreau & Fidrych, 1994).

Basic Concepts for Written Language Introduction

Once the students have learned a basic process for writing, it is time to write. This includes sentence formulation, paragraph formulation, grammar, punctuation, capitalization, and correct spelling to name a few considerations in the writing process. The following provides a list and explanation of the basic lessons and mechanics of writing that I have accumulated over the last several years. It provides a checklist that the student can use to target written language expression. These simple rules of writing will assist in a systematic strategy for the student to use at all times with written language.

Here Are the Basic Mechanics for Written Language

- If the paper is a one-paragraph essay to a writing prompt or answer to essay questions on a test, this will permit the student to have an introduction into the paragraph, which may be a restatement of the question (the main idea). The next three sentences will provide supporting details to the main idea with the remaining sentence being the conclusion.
- Each paragraph must have at least five sentences.
  - An introduction of the main idea of the paragraph
  - At least three details that support the main idea
  - A concluding sentence that summarizes the other statements
- The essay must have an introduction, body of development, and a conclusion.
  - If it is one paragraph, the introduction, body, and conclusion are in the same paragraph with the first sentence being the introduction; the next three sentences, the body; and the fifth sentence, the conclusion.
  - If it is a longer paper, the first paragraph with at least five sentences is the introduction.
    - The second, third, and fourth paragraphs are the body of development with each paragraph expanding on a thought.
    - The last paragraph is the conclusion.
- The first sentence MUST grab the reader's attention.
  - This is a good place to use an exclamatory statement, a simile, a metaphor, or an appropriate quotation.
  - The first sentence lets the reader know where the paper is heading. It must gain the reader's interest.

- o If it is a five-paragraph essay, the first sentence should peak the reader's interest in the topic.
- The introduction tells the main idea of the paper.
  - o If it is a one-paragraph paper, the main idea is the last sentence in the first paragraph. This also is referred to as the thesis statement. A thesis statement can be described as the key statement that tells about the content of the paper.
  - o If it is at least a five-paragraph paper, the first paragraph is the introduction with the last sentence being the thesis statement.
- The next three sentences or paragraphs develop the main idea.
- The conclusion tells what you just told and finishes with a final thought.
  - o If it is the conclusion of a one-paragraph essay, the conclusion is the final sentence.
  - o If it is a five-paragraph paper, the conclusion will be the second to last or last sentence in the final paragraph.
- Always use the same verb tense throughout the paper. If you started in present tense, the entire paper must be present tense.
  - o Papers should be written in present tense. This is especially true for a paper regarding literature because the student is currently reading the literature.
- Do not use "I" or "you" in the paper unless the teacher states that it is an informal paper.
  - o A formal paper is always written in the third person (one, he, she).
  - o One does not place their opinions unless requested by the teacher.
- Make sure to use complete sentences. A complete sentence has at least a subject (noun) and a predicate (verb) and relays a complete thought.
  - o If the student has used a conjunction (and, or, etc.) to join two thoughts together, then the next time a conjunction is used in that sentence, the student should consider using a period, and start the next sentence.
  - o FANBOYS: The coordinating conjunctions "for, and, nor, but, or, yet, so" are conjunctions that require a comma before the conjunction when joining two sentences (independent clauses) together. The subordinating conjunctions (after, although, as, as if, because, before, even if, even though, if, if only, rather than, since, that, though, unless, until, when, where, whereas, wherever, whether, which, and while) do not require a comma unless used in the beginning of a sentence as a subordinate clause.
- If a number is less than three digits, write it out (e.g., thirty-five).
- When to use commas:
  - o To separate two thoughts in the same sentence when using a FANBOY conjunction (I went to the store, and I bought bread.)
  - o To separate a dependent clause (In the morning, I went to the store.) (When John was finished with his work, he went outside.)

- To separate items in a series (bread, milk, and eggs). Always use a comma before "and" or "or" when listing items in a series.
- When using quotation marks
  - A comma goes before the quote begins and the punctuation mark goes inside the quotes. For example: John said, "I want to go to the movies."
  - The ending mark goes inside the ending quotation mark.

In conclusion, learning basic lessons of the writing process will provide a strategy in order to write a paper that is more organized and has good content. This also will provide a consistent strategy for the student to begin writing. Once the main framework of the paper is complete, the student can then concentrate on being descriptive in the writing.

Grammar Introduction

I had a student who came to see me the summer before his seventh grade year. His English teacher was going to work with him that summer as well to assist with increasing his understanding of parts of speech. After the first week of summer tutoring, this teacher announced that she would be unable to continue for the summer and asked if I would work on grammar with this student. The resource teacher of the student's school recommended using The Winston Grammar Program Basic Level (Erwin, 2007) and the Advanced Level (Erwin, 2005). I purchased the series and then thought, "How am I going to teach grammar?" As I have stated over and over again in this text, I told myself to go back to what the student already knows and build from there. Following are the steps used to increase this student's grammar knowledge and how we moved this knowledge into written expression. I have continued to use these same strategies with other students with great success.

Here's How to Assist With Understanding Grammar

- Start with what the student knows.
  The first piece of grammar that a student learns is what a noun is (a person, place, or thing). The second piece of grammar is what a verb is. The next step would be to expand on what the student knows.

Understanding Grammar Strategies

- Expand on nouns.
  - A noun can be common or proper.
    - Common noun = everyday words: man, house, ball

- Proper noun = a specific person, place or thing (Mr. Smith, Eiffel Tower, Toll House Cookies)
  - A noun can be used as the subject, direct object, indirect object, object of a preposition, pronoun, predicate nominative, or a noun of a direct address.
- Expand on verbs.
  - Action verbs (verbs that show action: run, walk, sit)
  - Verbs of being (am, is, are, was, were, be, being, been, become, seem)
  - Verbs used as a predicate (the main verb in the sentence that tells what the subject is doing)
- Introduce or review prepositions.
  - Prepositions include place, direction, and time.
    - Place prepositions include words such as in, on, at.
    - Direction prepositions include words such as under, over, right and left.
    - Time prepositions include words such as in, at, on, for, during, while.
  - A simple method to determine if a word is a preposition of place or direction is to place the potential preposition word in front of a phrase such as "the box."
- Introduce or review prepositional phrases (a group of words containing a preposition, a noun or pronoun, object of the preposition, and any modifiers of the object).
  - Introduce or review nouns as the object of the preposition.
- A sentence must have a subject (noun), predicate (verb), and a complete thought to be a sentence.
- Analyze sentences containing a subject, predicate, prepositional phrase (preposition and object of the preposition). For example:

The dog is inside the house.

  - "Dog" is the subject (the dog is the complete subject).
  - "is" is the verb or predicate.
  - "inside" is the preposition.
  - "the house" is the object of the preposition.
  - "inside the house" is the prepositional phrase.

I have found that once a student is able to identify these four parts of speech that it is easier to identify other parts of speech such as adjectives, adverbs, and direct and indirect objects.

- Adjectives (tells about the noun)
  - Which (tall boy)
  - What kind of (nice boy)
  - How many (two boys)
  - How much (little boy)

- Adverb (tells about the verb, adjective, or adverb)
  - Mostly end in –ly
  - Exceptions to –ly (very, not, here, there, too, also, never, always, ever)
  - Answers
    - When (tomorrow, often)
    - How (securely)
    - Where (down) (confusing because it is often the same words used as prepositions)
    - Why
    - To what extent (snow falls heavily)
- Conjunctions
  If a conjunction is used to join two complete sentences together, the sentence is then a compound sentence. A complex sentence has an independent clause joined by one or more dependent clauses. A compound/complex sentence has at least two independent clauses and one or more dependent clauses. Two types of conjunctions are used for joining dependent or independent clauses.
  - Coordinating conjunctions
    - Join two complete sentences together with and, but, for, yet, or, or nor
    - Require the use of a comma before the conjunction if joining two independent clauses
  - Subordinating conjunctions
    - Join two complete sentences together with as, because, then, that, even though, before, whenever
    - Do not require a comma before the conjunction if the subordinating clause is at the end of the sentence
    - If the subordinate clause is at the beginning of the sentence, then a comma is used

If the student can identify these parts of speech, he or she should be able to write complete sentences and avoid fragments and run-on sentences while writing. A fragment is defined as an incomplete sentence. A run-on is described as two or more sentences in a paragraph without appropriate punctuation or connecting words or incorrectly joined sentences that should be written separately or rewritten as a compound or complex sentence.

Here's Additional Grammar Information for Older Students

Older students may be required to use compound or complex sentences in their writing as described earlier. They also may be required to use similes, metaphors, and/or figurative language for further description. It is important to make sure that the older student understands the basic information that has been provided thus far. Without this understanding, this student may not be able to provide the more complex sentence structure or figurative language that is required. This section provides additional information regarding these areas for the older student.

Figurative Language Described

Figurative language is defined as describing something by comparing it with something else. There are several types of figurative language that may be required in a writing assignment of an older student.

- Imagery
  Descriptions of people or objects stated in terms of our senses. Example: The flowers were waving hello.

- Simile
  A figure of speech used to express a resemblance between things of different kinds usually formed with *like* or *as*. Example: It is as big as a house.

- Metaphor
  A figure of speech used to express a similarity between two ideas that are not usually used together. Example: The inside of the car was cavernous.

- Alliteration
  Repeated consonant or vowel sounds that occur at the beginning of words or within words. Example: Sally sells sea shells.

- Personification
  A figure of speech used to give the qualities of a person to an animal, an object, or an idea. It is a comparison that the author uses to show something in an entirely new light, to communicate a certain feeling or attitude toward it, and to control the way a reader perceives it. Example: Lightning danced across the sky.

- Onomatopoeia
  The use of words used to represent mimic sounds. They appeal to our sense of hearing and they help bring a description to life. Example: Crunch, crunch, crunch goes the candy bar.

- Hyperbole
  An exaggerated statement used to heighten effect. It is not used to mislead the reader, but to emphasize a point. Example: Several million

- Idioms
  Expressions used that have a meaning other than the separate words. Example: Clear as a bell

One method for adding figurative language would be to have the student complete the prewriting process using a graphic organizer. When this is completed, the student should look at each area that will be included in the paper and decide where figurative language would be appropriate. The sentence can be written during the prewriting process to include the figurative language.

In conclusion, written language expression requires a student to understand many language aspects. The student must be able to figure out the main idea and supporting details. He or she must have the vocabulary knowledge in order to form a descriptive sentence. Then the student has to be able to place these thoughts into grammatically correct sentences and in a logical order. Written language expression is a complex task with many underlying language requirements.

Remediation, Modifications, Accommodations, and Bypass Strategies Introduction

Students with written language expression disorders may require accommodations for written assignments. This could include modifications to assignments. It could also include the use of an assistive device.

Here Are Some Accommodations for Written Language

- Shortening assignments
- Changing the format of the assignment
- Increasing time to complete the assignment
- Providing untimed tests that require writing
- Grading on content of the work and then on the quality
- Avoiding negative reinforcement
- Allowing the student to turn in the assignment for feedback. Revisions accepted for grade. (I typically write the number of changes each sentence requires in front of the sentence and have the student attempt to find the errors. We then discuss the reason for the change.)
- Allowing the use of electronic devices or the computer for word processing and other writing software applications

Here's How to Use the Computer and Writing Software/Tools

Bypass tools include ways to develop ideas, brainstorm, and organize information for writing. Many software tools also include word prediction software, which recalls frequently used words by the student. Some also provide speech to text where the student speaks into a microphone and the assistive technology types it on the screen. Spell check and a thesaurus are available on the word-processing devices. Bypass strategies include the following:

- Teaching keyboarding skills: This is especially true for students who have fine-motor difficulties that make pencil-to-paper tasks more difficult.

- Using assistive computer programs for graphic organizers and outlining
  - Kidspiration®
    Kidspiration is for students from kindergarten until fifth grade. It uses idea maps to stimulate ideas about a topic, concept maps to link information together, webs for organization and prewriting. This program typically offers a free 30-day trial. (Inspiration Software, Inc., n.d.)
  - Inspiration®
    Inspiration is designed for students in 6th through 12th grade. This program provides the same visual strategies as Kidspiration. It provides more options for research and evaluation (Inspiration Software, Inc., n.d.).
  - Draft Builder
    This program provides a means for brainstorming, note taking, and writing drafts (Don Johnston Incorporated, n.d.).
  - NEO 2®
    This portable word processor (laptop) designed for writing replaces the Alphasmart laptop. The NEO 2 includes 387 writing lessons. It uses Google Docs to store, edit, and share documents. It is also wireless, which allows students to send their writing directly to their teacher (NEO Direct, n.d.).
  - Fusion® (http://www.writelearning.com)
    This portable word processor includes word prediction and writing prompts.
  - Fusion
    This portable word processor is offered from the same company as the Fusion. This laptop provides a keyboard mastery program and writing skills development including writing prompts and writing tips (Writer Learning, n.d.)
  - Apps for tablet devices and smart phones
    There are new note-taking applications being developed daily for use with tablet devices and smart phones. Here are a few examples:
    - Penultimate: This app is available from Cocoa Box Design.
    - Note Taker HD: This is available through Software Garden.
    - Use Your Handwriting Gold: This app is available through Gee Whiz Stuff (Wagner, 2010).
    - Essay Czar: This is an essay writing handbook for college and high school students.
    - Achievers Writing Center: It provides writing assistant and full editing services.
    - Ask Czarina: This app has a live editor to answer students' questions free of charge.
    - The Essay Writing Wizard: Essays can be submitted from this app.
    - ESL Essay Writing: This app is geared for English as Second Language Student (IPADMODO, 2011)

Editing Checklist

Once the student is writing successfully, a checklist can be used to review the components of the writing assignment that should be completed before the student turns it in to the teacher. This provides the student the means to check his or her own work before a grade is given.

Here's How to Use an Edit Checklist for Writing

Students need to be able to critically review their own writing once a draft is completed. The following checklist will provide students with a systematic approach for reviewing their writing.

- Check for capitalization.
  - Every sentence begins with a capital letter.
  - Proper names are always capitalized (a person's name, a place such as a city, state, name of building, name of place, etc.).
- Check for punctuation.
  - A comma is used before FANBOYS (for, and, nor, but, or, yet, so) conjunctions when they join two sentences together.
  - A comma is used to separate items in a series. A comma should go before the words *and* and *or* when used in a series.
  - A comma is placed before the open quotation marks for a quotation.
  - A comma is used after a dependent clause is used at the beginning of the sentence.
  - Quotation marks are used whenever quoting someone directly.
  - Ending punctuation is always used.
    - A period is used for declarative sentences (making a statement), imperative statements (commands), and an indirect question.
    - An exclamation point is used for exclamatory sentences. Exclamatory sentences show excitement.
    - A question mark is used for the end of a direct question.
- Check for complete sentences (subject, predicate, complete thought).
  - If more than one conjunction is used to join ideas together, it is a good idea to start a new sentence.
  - If a sentence goes more than one line, assess whether it is a run-on.
  - Compound sentences separate the independent clauses with a comma if it is joined by a coordinating conjunction and no comma if it is a subordinating conjunction.
  - Complex sentences contain an independent and a dependent clause. A comma is used if the dependent clause comes before the independent clause. It does not have a comma if it is after the independent clause.

- Check for verb tense.
    - The same verb tense should be used throughout the paper.
    - Papers are usually written in present tense.
- Check for subject and verb agreement.
- Write out numbers that are one or two digits.
- Use numerals for numbers that are three digits and greater.
- Check for:
    - Introduction
    - Body
    - Conclusion

Conclusion

Research studies verify that written language expression is difficult for many students. It is especially difficult for students with a language-based learning disability. Elementary students can be provided consistent strategies to develop writing skills. This includes ways to brainstorm ideas and organize the ideas using a web or other graphic organizers to determine the main idea of the paper and the details to support the main idea.

The same strategies should be continued and required for middle school and high school. By the upper elementary grades, if the student continues to struggle significantly with written expression, accommodations, modifications, or bypass strategies may need to be considered.

The ability to write in a logical, organized manner is crucial to academic success. Students need to be able to answer questions in writing to demonstrate comprehension of literature and subject-based curriculum. They must provide information in writing on a test for essay questions. They also must demonstrate the ability to plan and organize information for writing prompts and one-paragraph essays. In addition, students must develop the skills needed to write research-based papers. Written language expression is the culmination of many simultaneous and sequential skills with many of the skills being problematic for those students with a speech and/or language disorder.

References

Auman, M. (1999). Step Up to Writing [Computer program]. Dallas, TX: Cambium Learning, Inc.

Bishop, D., & Clarkson, B. (2003). Written language as a window into residual language deficits: A study of children with persistent and residual speech and language impairments. *Cortex, 39,* 215–237.

Carrow-Woolfolk, E. (1996). *Oral Written Language Scales (OWLS).* Bloomington, MN: AGS.

Dockrell, J., Lindsay, G., Connelly, V., & Mackie, C. (2007). Constraints in the production of written text in children with specific language impairments. *Exceptional Children, 73,* 147–164.

Don Johnston Incorporated. (n.d.). Draft Builder 6 [Computer program]. Retrieved January 21, 2011, from http://www.donjohnston.com

Erwin, P. (2005). *The Winston grammar program advanced level.* Battle Ground, WA: Precious Memories Educational Resources.

Erwin, P. (2007). *The Winston grammar program basic level.* Battle Ground, WA: Precious Memories Educational Resources.

Hammil, D., Brown, V., Larsen, S. (2009). *Test of Written Language 4.* Austin, TX: Pro-Ed.

Hresko, W., Herron, S., & Peak, P. (2001). *Test of Early Written Language TEWL-2* (Complete kit). Washington DC: Pro Education.

Inspiration Software, Inc. (n.d.). Inspiration 9: 6-12 [Computer program]. Retrieved January 22, 2011, from http://www.inspiration.com

Inspiration Software, Inc. (n.d.). Kidspiration K-5 [Computer program]. Retrieved January 22, 2011, from http://www.inspiration.com

IPADMODO. (2011, February 2). Retrieved February 17, 2011, from http://ipadmodo.com/10755/student-focused-apps-advance-writing-skills-and-improve-thinking-acumen/

Katz, L., Fallon, K., Blenkarn, K., Smith, M., John, J., Olszewski, K., et al. (2007). *Written language & the school-based speech-language pathologist: A national survey.* Paper presented at the American Speech-Language-Hearing Association National Convention, Boston, MA.

Lutkus, A., Weiner, A., Daane, M., & Jin, Y. (2003). *The nation's report card: Reading 2002, Trial Urban District Assessment* (NCES 2003-523). Washington, DC: U.S. Department of Education, Institute of Education Sciences, National Center for Education Statistics.

Moreau, M., & Fidrych, H. (1994). The Story Grammar Marker [Computer program]. Springfield, MA: Mindwing Concepts, Inc.

NEO Direct. (n.d.). NEO 2. Retrieved November 11, 2009, from http://www.neo-direct.com

Salahu-Din, D., Persky, H., & Miller, J. (2008). *The nation's report card: Writing 2007* (NCES 2008-468). Washington, DC: U.S. Department of Education, Institute of Education Sciences, National Center for Education Statistics.

Scott, C., & Windsor, J. (2000). General language performance measures in spoken and written narrative and expository discourse of school-age children with language learning disabilities. *Journal of Speech, Language, and Hearing Research, 43,* 324–339.

Singer, B. D. (1995). Written language development and disorders: Selected principles, patterns, and intervention possibilities. *Topics in Language Disorders, 16*(1), 83–98.

Singer, B. D., & Bashir, A. S. (2004). Developmental variations in writing composition skills. In C. A. Stone, E. R. Silliman, B. J. Ehren, & K. Apel (Eds.), *Handbook of language and literacy* (pp. 559–582). New York, NY: The Guilford Press.

Smith, J. O. (1993). Self-reported written language difficulties of university students with learning disabilities. *Journal of Postsecondary Education and Disability, 10*(3).

Wagner, M. (2010, July 6). *4 iPad apps for handwriting and idea-sketching.* Tool Talk. Retrieved February 16, 2011, from http://blogs.computerworld.com/16474/4_ipad_apps_for_hand_writing_and_idea_sketching

Wechsler, D. (2009). *Wechsler Individual Achievement Test III* (3rd ed.). Austin, TX: Pro-Ed.

Wolf Nelson, N., Barh, C., & Van Meter, A. (2004). *The writing lab approach to language instruction and intervention.* Baltimore, MA: Brookes.

Woodcock, R., McGrew, K., & Mather, N. (2001). *Woodcock-Johnson III-Tests of Achievement* (3rd ed). Rolling Meadows, IL: Riverside.

Writer Learning. (n.d.). Fusion and Writer. Retrieved January 22, 2011, from http://www.writerlearning.com/

7

Publishers Provide What?

Introduction

As I continue to work with students who have online access to resources from textbook publishers, I am amazed and excited about what is available for them and, in particular, for students with language-based learning disabilities. It is amazing to think that several high schools around the country no longer have textbooks but instead have laptops or tablet devices and students have access to all of their textbooks and assignments online (Collom, 2009). As I enter the username and password provided by the teachers of the students I see, I am excited as I navigate through each chapter, listen to each paragraph as I hit the speaker button, and click on the vocabulary words. I also click on icons that provide information on study skills and other icons that provide a section summary. The wealth of information being offered is phenomenal.

This chapter reviews many of the resources that are available from textbook publishers and discusses how these resources assist all students and, in particular, those with language-based learning disabilities. I have not listed specific publishers under what may be offered. Instead I suggest that you look at the publishers for the curriculum that is being used for the students you see and determine what may be available. I typically check with the classroom teachers for the textbook information as well as usernames and passwords. Teachers should have the access usernames and passwords for the textbooks they are using if resources are available online.

Here Are the Resources That Publishers Offer for Teachers

- Training and Development: Many publishers offer on-site and Web-based training for educators. This includes orientation to the new textbooks to teaching strategies.

- Interactive Presentation Tools: Many publishers provide interactive presentation tools including transparencies and PowerPoint presentations that teachers can use to teach particular lessons.

- Editable Teacher Resources: With these resources teachers can edit questions, create questions, and create different versions of worksheets, quizzes, and tests. This can assist educators in constructing tests based on differential instruction and students' current levels.

- Interactive Download Whiteboard: Many publishers offer digital software that can be used with a whiteboard. It includes downloadable audio and video to use in the classroom. This is exciting because this information can then be sent to students who are using laptops or specialized computers to assist with learning.

- Online Homework and Additional Practice: Teachers can assign homework, which students can access online. If a student needs additional practice for particular concepts, further practice may be available.

- Differential Instruction:
  - Multileveled readers: Material is presented based on the students' skills. These can be materials for those who are struggling to materials for those with advanced skills.
  - Multileveled worksheets: These worksheets go along with the multileveled materials that the students are using.
  - Leveled resources: These are additional resources from the publisher and recommended Internet sites based on the students' current levels.
  - Audio text: Online textbooks show a speaker or other symbol. If the student clicks on the speaker, the text will be read.

- Writing Prompts: These include possible topics based on the context of the information being provided.

- Graphic Organizers: Many publishers offer graphic organizers that can be downloaded or printed for the students.

- Suggested Reading Lists: These are additional readings that the teacher could assign to support the information currently being taught.

- Online Tests and Scorer: Students can take tests online, which are scored for the teacher, thus decreasing the time it takes the teacher to score the tests. The teacher can then review the results and decide if further learning is needed before moving on to a new section or topic. The teacher can use the suggested reading list or Internet links for further learning.

In summary, textbook publishers offer a variety of resources for educators. Teachers have so many teaching tools at their disposal that are within the curriculum being used by the schools.

Resources for Students

- Online Textbooks: Remembering to take the correct textbook home becomes unnecessary when students have access to their textbook online. They are ready to begin homework as long as they have the assignment written down or their teachers post them online. Parents no longer have to document that their student did not have the correct book or have to make the trip back to school to get the correct one. The need for backpack check also is no longer needed to ensure that the appropriate books are going home at the end of the day.

  Many of the ebooks also permit students to highlight details as they are reading. Some applications allow students to add notes as they read. With this application students can type in the main idea and supporting details next to the information in the text and then use the notes area to write a summary of the section as part of test preparation.

  If an ebook does not provide the resource for highlighting or taking notes, students can print the pages and then underline or highlight key words on those pages to increase reading comprehension.

- Audio: The information that follows may be available on audio. The section of the book where these items are located may include a speaker button, which, when pushed, presents the following information:
  - Sections
  - Speeches
  - Letters
  - Interviews
  - Music
  - News reports

  This will encourage students to listen and read at the same time in order to increase comprehension. It also provides students the opportunity to gain greater information and insight by paying attention to the additional information presented via audio.

- Reading Help:
  - Highlighted vocabulary words: Students can click on the vocabulary word as it is presented in the beginning of the chapter or in the actual section and make the vocabulary card at that time. The highlighted word also may be presented via audio, which would provide both auditory and reading to increase comprehension.
  - Section outline summaries: Students can click on an icon that provides a pop-up box with an outline of the key concepts presented in a particular section or lesson. This will assist them in understanding the main idea and supporting details.

- Textbook Companion: These are additional materials that students can use to increase learning of the information being studied.

- Study Skills: These are sometimes included between chapters. Study skills present strategies that are listed throughout the text. They would serve as a reminder of how to use the strategies that have been presented.

- Test-Taking Strategies: Publishers may offer supplemental information regarding test-taking strategies for classroom and standardized tests. This may be a section on the publishers' Web site or information in the specific text that includes specific strategies (e.g., review test format, types of questions, guidelines for grading) to prepare for the test. It also may include downloads with specific strategies to practice.

- Self-Tests and Quizzes: These allow students to quiz themselves and obtain immediate feedback regarding successful and missed items. They can serve as a great review to check and make sure that all pertinent information is in the notes. They also assess test readiness.

- Additional Practice: This provides students with more homework practice for information that they have not yet mastered.

- Additional Assistance From Publishers and Selected Online Resources: Publishers often have a link that will take students from the secured site back to the publishers' main site or to selected Internet sites. This will increase the students' knowledge base regarding a specific subject.

In summary, access to the many resources available for students provides the tools to increase academic success.

Here Are Some Advantages for Students With Language-Based Learning Disabilities

All students would benefit from the plethora of information that publishers now provide. Students with language-based learning disabilities would benefit further. The following list discusses some of those benefits.

- Assists students with reading all information presented: Being able to read along with the audio presentation may encourage students to review each page, thus increasing their understanding of the information being presented. It is easy to move from section to section by looking for the next speaker icon on the page. By listening to the text, the students also read and hear all of the words instead of misreading or skimming sections.

- Provides study skills, test-taking strategies, and organizational strategies: Often these skills are not intuitive for students with learning disabilities. Having the skills linked to what they are currently learning will assist students in learning new strategies. It also will increase the relevance of the strategies for the students.

- Reads the text: Students have two modalities of input to increase comprehension of the information: they can follow along in the text while it is presented online audibly.

- Provides information at the students' ability level: Leveled readers present the information at each student's current level to increase understanding of the material. The same content and vocabulary are presented but at a reading level appropriate for the student.

- Provides definitions for vocabulary in writing and audio: This encourages students to make their vocabulary cards as they click on each highlighted word because the definition pops up. They can also click on the speaker button and hear the word and definition.

- Provides section outline summaries: This provides students with the most important information regarding a section in the textbook such as the main idea and the supporting details. The students can then use this information to build Cornell Notes.

- Provides further clarification and information from publishers and online of content that is not included in the textbook: Many publishers offer additional information regarding the content presented through the textbook online or through recommended online sites.

- Provides quizzes to assess understanding of information: Students can study the information then quiz themselves. The online quiz grades the score as soon as students click the button after completing the items. This will provide them with immediate feedback so that they know what information they need to study more in depth before the examination.

- Increases understanding of content: Students are receiving the information through two modalities by being able to read along as the text is read. This will assist the students' understanding of the information.

In conclusion, there are so many online resources available through textbook publishers for teachers and students to enhance learning. The additional information and resources that are available will assist students with any learning differences, providing them tremendous opportunities to learn information. Students with language-based learning disabilities will greatly benefit from all the additional resources—from test-taking strategies, study skills, and organizational strategies to enhanced learning through audio input to section summaries. From the struggling reader to the student with difficulty with comprehension, these additional resources offer the support for academic success.

Reference

Collom, L. (2009, August 27). Poston Butte high-school students go digital. *The Arizona Republic*. Retrieved April 24, 2011, from http://www.azcentral.com/arizonarepublic

8

Classroom Strategies

Introduction

Everyone likes to be successful. However, it is easier to be successful when the expectations are known and are consistent. Imagine a classroom environment where regardless of grade level or teacher, the expectations and strategies used are always the same. For instance, when a math word problem is presented, the same steps are followed and documented each time; when a book report is due, the same format is used to gather information from the book; or when a project is due, the same planning and writing format is required. I have had the opportunity to see this work in the education environment. I was able to discharge students with significant language-based learning disabilities because of this consistency. The students were learning and thriving without additional intervention.

Response to Intervention (RTI) calls for evidence-based practices. RTI also calls for recognizing when a student is struggling and using evidence-based practices to quickly make changes to the teaching strategies being used. There is substantial evidence regarding the use of graphic organizers and mnemonics for students with language-based learning disabilities (Kim & Vaughn, 2004). Imagine an educational environment where consistency is the key regardless of class, teacher, or grade level!

I know that this would be the ideal environment. Many of us may not have the authority to implement such systemwide changes; therefore, we have to look at what can we do to make students successful within our scope of practice in our given environments.

This chapter begins with an overview of what a consistent environment for academic success of all students could potentially provide. A consistent environment means that regardless of academic subject, grade level, or educator the same strategies are employed for optimal learning. As stated previously, many of us may not have the ability to make sweeping changes in our current environments. It is hoped that some of the strategies introduced could be incorporated into the academic environment that meet your state and local district standards. These strategies are excellent for RTI Tier I classroom instruction,

RTI Tier 2 small group instruction, as well as RTI Tier 3 individual instruction. This chapter reviews strategies that can be used across the curriculum as well as reasonable accommodations and the purpose of the accommodations. These accommodations or modifications are in line with the Individuals with Disability Education Act 2004 (IDEA) as well as Section 504 of the Americans with Disabilities Amendments Act (ADAA) as described in the introductory chapter of this book.

Introduction to a Consistent Environment

In most states, speech-language pathologists in the school setting have exceptionally large caseloads and workloads. With the addition of RTI, many therapists question how they can handle their current workload, be involved in the classroom, and be part of the RTI team. This section provides a culmination of all of the strategies presented throughout the other chapters of this book and demonstrates how these techniques can be used for all students to be successful. The goal of implementing these strategies across the academic setting hopefully will lead to increased academic success for all students and decrease therapists' caseloads due to consistent expectations and increased knowledge and performance for all students. The suggestions for a consistent environment are separated into prekindergarten/kindergarten, first/second grade, and third grade forward.

Prekindergarten/Kindergarten

Prekindergarten classrooms should have a strong, organized focus on preliteracy and early literacy skills. As discussed in chapter 3, this includes activities for phonological awareness, phoneme awareness, alphabetic principle, auditory short-term memory, and sequencing. Many children will need daily reinforcement of activities in these areas.

Here are some possible examples that could be included to assist students with their language skills.

Schedule Boards

A schedule board could be placed on the wall to provide students with a visual schedule in order to know what is expected throughout the school day. It should include the word and a picture to represent the activity. This schedule can then be printed and sent home, providing communication to the parents each day. The section on the right can be used to write a brief description (or typed to be placed on the school's Web site) so that parents can discuss what occurred at school that day (Table 8–1).

This schedule board also serves as a visual reminder to assist students with the daily events. It provides a visual cue to assist them when the teacher gives a direction. They can use the visual cue to understand and remember (auditory short-term memory) what they are supposed to do. Many students with language disorders demonstrate difficulty with sequencing, which limits their ability to discuss events that have occurred. This

Table 8–1. Prekindergarten Schedule Sample.

Group Meeting	Calendar/Weather: A consistent song that presents the days of the weeks and months of the year is sung everyday as well as counting the days of the month that are completed. ABC + sounds: The teacher says the letter and students provide the body/hand movements and sounds that go with the letter.
Story Time	All stories presented have rhyming to increase understanding of word families, nursery rhymes, or fairy tales. The teacher asks questions while reading for the students to develop auditory memory, sequencing, vocabulary, and critical thinking skills (what will happen next, why do you think that happened). When the story is completed, the students participate in an activity to demonstrate understanding of the main idea, the details to support the main idea, and the sequence of the story.
Craft Time	The students must listen and follow the teacher's directions (auditory memory and sequencing) in order to complete the craft.
Math	Math programs for prekindergarten can include math concepts such as one, one more, all, and none. A math program for kindergarten usually includes manipulatives as well as a visual system.
Computer Time	Computer time usually provides educational software that reinforces what the students are learning. If a student needs additional phonemic awareness assistance, programs such as Earobics® could be used during this time to increase phonological awareness, discrimination, and processing.
ABC **Language Arts**	(Kindergarten) Researched-based curriculum usually includes phonics, phonetically regular words, and high-frequency words.
Writing/Journal	Students could have a journal in which write everyday. It is wonderful to see the progress in phonics, spelling, and sentence formation by the end of the year.
Free Time	Centers should be organized with a purpose. This may include creative play, age-appropriate books, sensory play (tactile, propioceptive, vestibular).

picture format allows parents to know what was discussed in morning meeting to what the students had for snack. Students can then look at the picture in order to sequence the day's events in the right order, and parents know if the information being provided is accurate. Parents also can provide hints to their student for more information.

Visual Reminders for Behavior

Classroom rules, stated positively, should also be posted on the wall with pictures to represent the rules. Rules may include: Feet on the floor. Sit with your legs criss crossed. Hands to your side. These also can be placed on a strip and laminated to place on the students' desks. It is amazing how these simple visual reminders will impact classroom behavior, which also is a part of RTI. In addition, it is much easier to learn if students are sitting quietly and attending.

Phonological Awareness, Phoneme Awareness, and the Alphabet Principle

- Phonological Awareness: At the prekindergarten/kindergarten level, a phonological awareness program could include the following:
  - ○ Segmenting a sentence into words: Students must understand that sentences are made up of individual words before they can understand that each word is made up of syllables then specific sounds. See Table 3–3 for examples of some simple sentences for this task.
  - ○ Segmenting words into syllables: At this age, how many claps a word has sometimes has more meaning. See Table 3–4 for examples of words with one to four syllables.
  - ○ Identifying individual sounds in words: At the prekindergarten level, students often identify the first sound and maybe the last sound. As they enter kindergarten, they begin to identify the vowel sound in the middle. This is typically short vowel sounds.
  - ○ Identifying and producing rhyming words: This important skill is needed for students to understand onset and rhymes for future word families as well as patterns in words that are similar. Chapter 3 provides specific activities that can be used. See Table 3–2 for examples of pairs of words that can be used for rhyming activities.
  - ○ Blending sounds to make words: This activity assists students with hearing and understanding individual sounds that make up a word.
- Phonemic Awareness and the Alphabetic Principle: I used to use a sound/symbol program that introduced one sound or symbol at a time. After spending time in prekindergarten and kindergarten classrooms, I found that using the alphabet and visual cues enabled students to learn the sounds and associated symbols much quicker. So I switched my approach and now go through the alphabet, adding specific hand signals every time. I do this at least 2 or 3 times in an hour session. Please refer to Table 3–5 for suggestions of hand signals that can be used. I prefer an alphabet border that does not have pictures associated with the letter. This often leads to the picture instead of the sound being associated with the letter. I then add hand signals for other sounds such as long vowels, digraphs, and diphthongs when we reach that level of phonological awareness and alphabetic principle.

In conclusion, prekindergarten and kindergarten students can benefit from an organized approach for learning. Regardless of the curriculum that is being used, a structure that includes consistent teaching strategies can assist all students at this level. This lays the foundation for the consistent environment that will continue throughout their educational career.

First and Second Grades

Research studies have found that there are six basic vowel patterns that students need to master in order to be efficient readers (Blachman & Tangel, 2008; VoWac, n.d.). These include:

- closed syllable as in "cat"
- consonant -le syllable as in "ta/ble"
- open syllable as in "me"
- vowel team syllable as in "read" (two vowels go walking and the first one does the talking or vowel teams)
- vowel-consonant-e syllable as in "cake" (magic e or silent e)
- r-controlled syllable as in "barn" and "bird"

This provides the basis for understanding phonics for reading and spelling and should be considered when planning strategies to be used with the curriculum.

- Phonological Awareness for First and Second Grades: By this time, the students should understand rhymes, phoneme awareness, the alphabetic principle; identify the initial, medial, and final sounds of one-syllable words; as well as identify syllables in words. A phonological awareness program in the first and second grades now can be combined with a phonics program, spelling, and a reading program. Activities may include:
  - Segmenting words into individual sounds: Students should continue to target breaking words down to their individual sounds.
  - Blending sounds to make words: Once they can segment words into their individual sound, students can blend those sounds together to make words. Reading and writing are now added to this activity as well as phonics rules to explain the symbols that go with the specific sounds.
  - Identifying and producing rhyming words: This skill now can be used to understand word families (at, cat, bat, hat). Phonics rules can be added for more difficult word families (-ind, -ould, -ome).
- Spelling: The foundation for successful reading and writing continues to be built at these grade levels. Spelling lists can continue to reinforce the patterns that are being taught. Students are not always intuitive regarding what pattern is being presented. The teacher or speech-language pathologist is encouraged to discuss the pattern with the students.

- High-Frequency Words: High-frequency words are typically added to spelling tests during these grades. Many high-frequency words have little meaning to students (the, a, some, come, would, could). Meaning should be applied to these words in order to increase storage strength for reading and writing.

- Vocabulary: Again as stated earlier, it is important to make sure that students understand the vocabulary words that are being presented. Understanding the words and any multiple meanings will support auditory and reading comprehension. Remember that if a student has a word-finding disorder, retrieval strength needs to be targeted in addition to storage strength of vocabulary words (German, 2007). Please refer to chapter 5.

As stated in chapter 5, Across the Curriculum, the folded note cards should be introduced at this time for the spelling words and high-frequency and vocabulary words. The format for these cards, listed in chapter 5, should be introduced. This begins the use of consistent strategies throughout the grade levels.

The use of the folded card or typed-on shipping size labels will continue for spelling and vocabulary throughout the students' academic career regardless of subject matter, teacher, or grade level.

Third Grade Forward

Once the students are on their way to fluent reading, consistent strategies for learning should be introduced. These are the same strategies that can be used throughout high school and into higher education. They include strategies such as highlighting key words in written directions and paragraphs, webs, Venn diagrams, Cornell Notes, book report format, and format for math story problems. These strategies are introduced in chapter 5. This section focuses on how these can be used consistently in the academic setting.

Webs

When discussing a story that has been read, the teacher can introduce webbing while discussing the main idea and supporting details. The main idea would be placed in the center circle of the web with the details in circles around it. A circle also can be added for a conclusion (how the story ended). As students progress, setting, plots, characters, conflict, and conflict resolution can be added.

Students can use the webs if a writing assignment follows the story or for any other writing assignments. Again, regardless of grade level, subject, or teacher, students would be expected to always use a web for organizing thoughts regarding a story or for any written assignment. This will assist them with any essays on classroom or standardized tests and serve as the prewriting requirement. If a student uses a program such as Inspiration, the web can be automatically converted to an outline if required for an assignment. For the older student who is required to complete projects, the web can be used to organize the requirements of the teacher to make sure that all the necessary information is included (Inspiration 9: 6-12, n.d.).

T Charts

T charts are perfect for comparing (similarities) or contrasting (differences). The first item that is being compared or contrasted goes on the left side of the "T" with the second topic on the right side. This provides a visual organizer so that if the student then needs to write a compare/contrast paper regarding the two items being compared or contrasted, the information is organized to assist in writing a more organized paper.

Venn Diagrams

Venn diagrams provide a great visual support for comparing and contrasting two or three concepts. This visual support provides a consistent means of organizing thoughts. Information that is the same is placed in the section that overlaps in the middle with the contrasting information placed on each side of the overlapping area. This provides a visual strategy to organize information. This also should assist students if a written assignment then follows.

Cornell Notes

Although webs can be used for note taking, I typically introduce Cornell Notes (see chapter 5 for an example) by fourth or fifth grade. This provides a way to take notes on more in-depth information such as Social Studies or Science. It is a strategy that can be used through higher education. The left side of the paper is a smaller column where the main idea, a picture, or questions can be written. The right column is where students take notes supporting the main idea.

Written Directions and Paragraph-Length Materials

As students increase their reading skills they will be required to follow written directions. Next the strategy for following written directions is introduced. The students should:

1. read the direction
2. read the direction a second time and underline the key words in the direction
3. follow the direction
4. go back and reread only the key words and make sure that all parts of the direction were followed
5. place a check mark above the section

Many students often do not read the directions because they assume that they understand what they are supposed to do. This technique requires them to read the direction because the teacher will see that the key words are underlined and checked off. This will ensure that the students are completing all parts of a direction and are not missing points due to incomplete work versus knowledge. This strategy will assist students with classroom test taking as well as standardized test taking. As they advance in grade level, this strategy also provides the foundation for reading information regarding projects that require specific steps and specific information to be reported.

This same strategy is used for following paragraph-length information as well as important information provided in a text. For paragraph-length information, students will need to determine the important information because not every sentence is important. After they ascertain the important sentences, then key words in those sentences can be highlighted. Products such as highlighting tape and erasable highlighters are available to highlight in textbooks. Highlighting tape peels back off easily and can be reused. One drawback of the tape is that it is difficult to highlight only important words. There also are erasable highlighters that can be used on text print. These highlight like a highlighter but erase easily. The ultimate goal is increased reading comprehension.

Written Language Expression

Written expression often is difficult for many students with or without language disabilities. Many students do not demonstrate proficiency by the time they leave high school (Salahu-Din, Persky, & Miller, 2008). Students with language-based learning disorders may demonstrate even greater difficulty. In order to be successful with written expression, students must be able to retrieve the words they know and be able to spell (phonics) those they do not know. They must formulate thoughts regarding what to write, organize the information, and then write. Students with word-finding difficulties will often write short, choppy sentences and reduced content. Students with receptive and expressive language disorder will demonstrate decreased vocabulary comprehension and expression. They may also demonstrate difficulties with developing content as well as using figurative language (similes, metaphors, expressions, etc.) in order to write an in-depth paper.

1. Teach the students to always use the following strategy for written expression:
   a. Choose a topic, if applicable.
   b. Research the topic.
   c. Generate a list of words that pertain to that topic.
   d. Place into categories the items from the list.

   EXAMPLE: Basketball

1	court	3	uniforms
1	ball	3	shoes
1	backboard	3	mouth guard
1	net	2	scoring
2	2 points	2	3 points
2	free throws		

   The information can then be used to establish a web to organize the information for writing a paragraph or a paper.

2. Assist the students with using webs, T charts, or Venn diagrams consistently to organize ideas.

3. Help students with writing complete sentences.
   If a web is used, each bubble from the web becomes at least one complete sentence. The first sentence is from the middle bubble, which is the main idea. Each detail that comes from the bubbles surrounding the main idea becomes at least one complete sentence. The last bubble should represent the conclusion. For a paper, the bubbles are the main idea and detail of each paragraph. The information written in the bubble for the main idea is usually the thesis statement or the last sentence in the introductory paragraph that explains the content of the paper.

   If a student is using a T chart or a Venn diagram, he or she should choose one section and completely develop the information in that section. Each section should follow in the same manner.

Math

A format for following math word problems should be introduced as soon as the math curriculum begins to challenge the students to complete math story problems. Many textbooks provide a strategy to use for solving word problems. This is usually provided the first time that word problems are introduced. Once the format is introduced, the students should continue to use this strategy ongoing. Students should always show the steps in solving the word problem. The following steps are what should be recorded on the paper. This strategy takes the underlining directions strategy and includes a couple more steps in order to gain the necessary information to solve the program.

- Read the problem carefully.
- Read the problem again.
  - Underline important words.
  - The sentence that begins with "What" tells you what you need to solve.
- Look for key words that should also be underlined (Table 8–2).
- Associate numbers with important information and write down that information; for example, a piece of property valued at $55,000 (property value = 55,000).
- Identify a starting point based on what the question is asking.
- Solve the problem.
- Reread to make sure you answered the question that is being asked (Table 8–3).

Use strategies to assist students in memorizing important functions (hand gestures and mnemonics).

- Hand gestures: In our study group, one student showed the group hand gestures that her math teacher taught them to memorize order of operations (parentheses,

Table 8–2. Math Key Words

English	Math
amounts to, total	equals
times, product	multiplication
less than, decreased by, reduced by, fewer than, minus	subtraction
by, total, in all, together with, combined with, more than, sum	add
half of, a quarter of, etc.	divide

Table 8–3. Math Story Problems Checklist

☐ Read the problem carefully.

☐ Read the problem again.

☐ Underline important words.

☐ Find what you are solving for (will probably start with "What").

☐ Associate numbers with important information and write down that information; e.g., a piece of property valued at $55,000 (property value = 55,000).

☐ Solve the problem.

☐ Reread to make sure you answered the question that is being asked.

exponents, multiply, divide, add, and subtract—left to right, left to right). Two weeks later, another student was solving math problems that required understanding order of operations. So the first student taught the second student the hand signals. The interesting point goes back to consistency among all of the educators. Both students were in the same grade at the same school but with different math teachers, so one student learned this great way to memorize the order of operations, and the other student did not and was still struggling with the concepts.

- Mneumonics: In staying with the same example, order of operations (parentheses, exponents, multiply, divide, add and subtract) also can be memorized by using the following:

  ○ PEMDAS

  ○ Please excuse my dear Aunt Sally

Lastly, using graph paper will assist students in keeping numbers properly aligned in order to complete the operations needed. Students should always be required to show their work. This will assist them with keeping information organized as well as show them a way to review if the answer is incorrect.

In conclusion, a consistent environment will lead to clear expectations of all students and greater success for all students. I am fortunate to work with a small school that provides the preceding framework across the grade levels. As I met with this school staff recently, more teachers have been added due to increased enrollment. Different teaching methods are being introduced, thus a move away from the consistent teaching strategies that worked so beautifully.

The RTI process calls for evidence-based teaching. Research has demonstrated that students require excellent phonological awareness skills for literacy skills. Research also shows us that the use of mnemonics and graphic organizers lead to greater academic success. There are many strategies that can be introduced in the classroom and through RTI Tier I and Tier II regardless of grade level, academic setting, teacher, or curriculum. This consistency at Tier I may be enough to assist those struggling learners to be successful.

It also is important to remember that students with a learning disability may spend more time than other students to complete homework assignments. So if educators give homework that they think should only take 30 minutes to complete, they should consider that these students who learn differently may require double that to complete the assignment. The following provides specific accommodations and modifications for learning difficulties typically seen with specific speech and language diagnoses. Some students will continue to require modifications and accommodations to their curriculum in order to be successful.

Accommodations for Students Introduction

Students who demonstrate little progress as they move through the tiers of RTI may be referred for evaluation and possible services through special education. As part of the individual education plan (IEP), accommodations should be considered based on the results of the strategies attempted through RTI and the results of the evaluation.

Here's How Accommodations Can Assist a Student

Environmental Adaptations

- Classroom audio system: Millet (2008) summarized research regarding the use of sound field systems for students. The following information supports the use of audio systems in the classroom:
  - Higher incidence of ear infections and related hearing loss in young children
  - Immature listening skills related to neuromaturation that continues into adolescents

- Poor classroom acoustics
- Signal-to-noise ratio in a typical classroom (Acceptable level: 35dBA)
- Noise levels: 65–75 dB in kindergarten classrooms; 55–65 dB in elementary classrooms; and 60–70 dB in high school classrooms

The benefits of using classroom audio systems are:

- Improved scores on dictated spelling
- Increased standardized test scores
- Greater literacy gains
- Improved attention
- Significant increase in phonological awareness when instruction was coupled with amplification
- Decreased referral rate for special education services (MARRS project summarized in Millet's report showed a 40% decrease in referrals after 5 years of using sound field systems)

- Preferential seating
  - Close to where the teacher provides instruction
  - Away from distractions
    - Noisy students
    - Open doors and windows
    - Pencil sharpeners
    - Buzzing fluorescent light
- Preteach/prelearn
  - Provide assignments at least one day before presented in class.
  - Provide PowerPoint presentations and lecture notes at least one day before presented in class.
- Supplemental visual material
  - Visual phonics cues on desk or board
  - Touch Math or other visual math strategies
  - Hundreds Chart for sequencing numbers
  - Pictures for behavior expectations
- Provide textbooks and books assigned for reading on audio.
- Allow extended time to complete assignments and tests.
- Allow extra breaks.
- Reduce homework requirement.
- Provide project and assignment information in writing.
  - Use online resources to provide project specifications and deadlines as well as assignments and tests schedule.
  - Write key words for directions on the board; for example, math, pg 5, 1–5.

- o Use a visual schedule of the day's events.
- Repeat directions and instructions.
- Have the student repeat directions.
- Assign a peer buddy.
  - o Permit the student to ask this peer buddy for clarification on assignments. This should be a peer buddy chosen by the teacher.
  - o Provide a copy of the students notes (especially if using a consistent note-taking method that will benefit the student).
- Provide a daily or weekly study plan.
- Provide copies of teacher's lectures, PowerPoint presentations, or smart board notes. Provide these at least the day before the information is given in class if possible so that the student can prelearn.
- Write the main ideas of the lesson on the board.
- Provide information regarding learning that will occur the next day so the student can prelearn. The student should:
  - o be encouraged to preread assignments for the next day
  - o take notes on what will be taught
  - o only take notes during the lecture of content that is not included in the notes previously taken
- Provide assignment notebook and backpack check.
- Inform the student about availability of assistive technology.
  - o Echo Smartpen—This device records and links audio to what students write. It has an infrared camera that can film the teacher. There also is a microphone to pick up the teacher's voice and a speaker and headphone adapter to play back classroom information to make sure that notes are complete. The Pulse Smartpen® also permits students to download the information to a computer. This allows the student who is taking notes but may get behind or not recall all of the important information a way to go back and listen to the information again (Livescribe, n.d.).
  - o NEO 2—The NEO 2 is a word-processing laptop that integrates with white boards, projectors, and classroom computers. The teacher can send lecture notes directly to the students' NEO 2 laptops so that they have the additional information that they may have not recalled during class (NEO, n.d.).
- Return written assignments with suggestions for changes.
- Call on the student as soon as he or she raises the hand.
- Prepare the student for when you will call on him or her for an oral answer.
- Provide extended test-taking time:
  - o For classroom testing
  - o For standardized testing

- Adapt a test-taking format.
  - Use true/false.
  - Use multiple choice.
  - Provide a word bank for fill-in-the-blank or open-ended questions.
- Reduce the amount of different tests given in one day.
- For exams:
  - Allow extra test-taking time.
  - Provide testing in a small group.
  - Provide a professional to make sure that students understand the written directions.
  - Read test items to the students.
  - Permit the students to review and change incorrect test responses on classroom tests before the final grade (Table 8–4).

Table 8–4. Accommodations Checklist

ACCOMMODATIONS
☐ Classroom audio system

☐ Preferential seating
• Close to where the teacher provides instruction
• Away from distractions
  ○ Noisy students
  ○ Open doors and windows
  ○ Pencil sharpeners
  ○ Buzzing fluorescent light

☐ Preteach/prelearn • Provide assignments at least one day before presented in class. • Provide PowerPoint presentations and lecture notes at least one day before presented in class
☐ Supplemental visual material • Visual phonics cues on desk or board • Touch Math or other visual math strategies • Hundreds Chart for sequencing numbers • Pictures for behavior expectations
☐ Provide textbooks and books assigned for reading on audio.
☐ Allow extended time to complete assignments and tests.
☐ Allow extra breaks. • Reduce homework requirement.

Table 8–4. *continued*

- ☐ Provide project and assignment information in writing.
    - Use online resources to provide project specifications and deadlines as well as assignments and tests schedule.
    - Write key words for directions on the board; e.g., math, pg 5, 1–5.
    - Use a visual schedule of the day's events.
- ☐ Repeat directions and instructions.
- ☐ Have the student repeat directions.
- ☐ Assign a peer buddy.
    - Permit the student to ask this peer buddy for clarification on assignments. This should be a peer buddy chosen by the teacher.
    - Provide a copy of the student's notes (especially if using a consistent note-taking method that will benefit the student).
- ☐ Provide a daily or weekly study plan.
- ☐ Provide copies of teacher's lectures, PowerPoint presentations, or smart board notes.
- ☐ Write the main ideas of the lesson on the board.
- ☐ Provide information regarding learning that will occur the next day so the student can prelearn. The student should:
    - be encouraged to preread assignments for the next day
    - take notes on what will be taught
    - only take notes during the lecture of content that is not included in the notes previously taken
- ☐ Provide assignment notebook and backpack check.
- ☐ Inform the student about availability of assistive technology.
    - Echo Smartpen
    - NEO 2 word-processing laptop
- ☐ Return written assignments with suggestions for changes.
- ☐ Call on student as soon as he or she raises the hand.
- ☐ Prepare the student for when you will call on him or her for an oral answer.
- ☐ Provide extended test-taking time:
    - For classroom testing
    - For standardized testing
- ☐ Adapt a test-taking format.
    - Use true/false.
    - Use multiple choice.
    - Provide a word bank for fill-in-the-blank or open-ended questions.
- ☐ Reduce the amount of different tests given in one day.
- ☐ For exams:
    - Allow extra test-taking time.
    - Provide testing in a small group.
    - Provide a professional to make sure that students understand the written directions
    - Read test items to the students.
    - Permit the students to review and change incorrect test responses on classroom tests before the final grade.

Consistency Across Grades and Educators Checklist

Table 8–5 offers a checklist of the information presented in this chapter. It provides a quick reference while working toward a consistent environment or making accommodations for specific students.

Table 8–5. Across Grade Level and Educators Checklist

PREKINDERGARTEN/KINDERGARTEN

☐ Consistent Schedule
• Group Meeting
  ○ Calendar
  ○ Weather
  ○ ABC and sounds

☐ Story Time • Use books with a purpose (letter and sound, word family, concepts) • Use questions about the book to build auditory memory, sequencing, vocabulary, and critical thinking • Use an activity to resequence story
☐ Language Arts (Kindergarten) • Structured phonemic awareness program • Structured phonological awareness program • Introduction to the alphabetic principle
☐ Craft • Require the students to follow step-by-step instructions to complete the craft.
☐ Math • Prekindergarten   ○ Concepts (more, less, one, one more, all, some, rest) • Kindergarten ○ Introduce a math program such as TouchMath (Innovative Learning Concepts, n.d.)

☐ Computer
• Programs with a purpose
  ○ Phonological awareness programs
  ○ Phonics program

☐ Writing/Journal • Introduce and require webs to organize thoughts (may be with pictures at this point)

☐ Free time
• Organize centers for specific purposes
  ○ Creative play
  ○ Building concepts
  ○ Support other information learned throughout the day

Table 8–5. *continued*

FIRST AND SECOND GRADES

☐ Continue strong phonological awareness and phonics program
  • Spelling words should be based on the phonic rule being taught not specific subject vocabulary

☐ High-frequency words: Make sure students understand the meaning of the words

☐ Vocabulary building based on subject specific vocabulary
  • Introduce a consistent method of using note cards for vocabulary practice

THIRD GRADE AND BEYOND

☐ Webs. These are used for:
  • understanding the main idea and supporting details
  • subject-based understanding
  • written expression organization
    ○ After the basic web is completed, add specific vocabulary
    ○ Metaphors/similes
    ○ Greater descriptions

☐ T charts
  • Compare
  • Contrast

☐ Venn diagrams
  • Compare and contrast
  • Similarities and differences

☐ Cornell Notes (by fourth or fifth grade) for note taking

☐ Written Directions and Paragraph-Length Information
  • Highlight/underline key words in directions
  • Highlight/underline paragraph-length information

☐ Written Expression
  • Organize thoughts
    ○ Choose a topic, if applicable
    ○ Research the topic
    ○ Generate a list of words that pertain to that topic
    ○ Place into categories the items from the list
  • Web thoughts
  • Use complete sentences with description (adjectives, adverbs, similes, metaphors)

☐ Math
  • Consistent steps for following math story problems
  • Consistent strategies to memorize information
  • Graph paper for organization of problems
  • Always show work

Conclusion

I remember going to college and being so excited that I could write and highlight in my textbooks and write notes in the margins. I remember how the yellow highlighted information caught my eye when I would review the information. I remember attempting new ways of studying because of being able to use my texts differently. I now think back to how much easier it would have been if I would have gone to college knowing the strategies that I know today as well as having the tools that are now available to our students. I have had so many parents say the same thing. I know that as individual professionals we may have little impact regarding implementing consistent environments for all of our students, but maybe collectively we can provide our students with strategies that will make ongoing learning easier across the curriculum.

References

Blachman, B., & Tangel, D. (2008). *Road to reading: A program for preventing and remediating reading difficulties.* Baltimore, MA: Paul H. Brookes.

Earobics. (n.d.). *A research driven multisensory learning solution.* Retrieved October 11, 2009, from http://www.earobics.com

German, D. (2007). *Dual-focus vocabulary instruction for word finding, meanings, and retrieval strategies.* Paper presented at the American Speech-Language-Hearing Association National Convention, Boston, MA.

Innovative Learning Concepts. (n.d.). Touch-Math. Retrieved October 2, 2009, from http://www.touchmath.com

Inspiration Software, Inc. (n.d.). Inspiration 9: 6-12 [Computer program]. Retrieved February 6, 2009, from http://www.inspiration.com

Livescribes. (n.d.). Livescribe's smart pen. Retrieved February 19, 2011, from http://www.livescribe.com/en-us/smartpen/echo/

Kim, A., & Vaughn, S. (2004). Graphic organizers and their effects on the reading comprehension of students with LD: A synthesis of research. *Journal of Learning Disabilities, 37*(2), 105–118. Retrieved December 6, 2010, from www.asha.org

Millett, P. (2008). Sound field amplification research summary. Ontario, Canada: York University. Retrieved February 18, 2011, from http://gofrontrow.com/files/documents/research/sound-field-amplification-research-summary.pdf

NEO Direct. (n.d.). NEO 2. Retrieved February 19, 2011, from http://www.neo-direct.com

Salahu-Din, D., Persky, H., & Miller, J. (2008). *The nation's report card: Writing 2007* (NCES 2008–468). Washington, DC: U.S. Department of Education, Institute of Education Sciences, National Center for Education Statistics.

VoWac Publishing Co. (n.d.). *Phonics.* Retrieved October 2, 2009, from http://www.vowac.com/Programs/Phonics.aspx

9

Strategies for Home

Introduction

Parents play a crucial role is assisting their child to become more independent with the strategies that will increase academic success. This includes participating in therapy when possible, completing therapy assignments, helping with school homework, or working to increase particular academic skills. If the parents do not have an opportunity to participate in therapy, I provide information at the onset of therapy that explains the strategies that will be used. This provides a resource for the parents to use to assist their student at home. I always attempt to address my goals in therapy through the students' homework or an academic subject that we can prelearn for the next day's class.

With Response to Intervention (RTI), parent involvement starts at the very beginning. Each tier of RTI specifies the role of the parent.

1. Tier 1 Intervention
   - Notify the parents that their child has been identified through assessment as needing intervention.
   - Conduct a parent/teacher conference.
     ○ Offer strategies and materials for home instruction.

2. Tier 2 Intervention
   - Continue to send home reports and continuous progress monitoring data reviewed by the team.
   - Involve parents in team meetings to review progress and make instructional decisions.
     ○ Provide information from the meeting in writing to the parents.

3. Tier 3 Intervention
   - Send form letter home.
   - Obtain consent for individual evaluation.
   - Conduct follow-up call to address parent questions.

Home Strategies for Preliteracy Skills Introduction

A child's first teacher is the parent. Parents can set the stage for learning to be fun. My favorite gift to give to parents of a new baby is cardboard books. They probably often think that it is a silly gift for such a young baby. My implied message is to start reading to their child regardless of the age. The way parents interact with their children through books, singing, and pointing out fascinating objects in the environment opens up the world of learning and lays the foundation of skills needed for future academic success.

Here's How Parents Can Assist Their Child With Preliteracy Skills

- Read, read, read.
  - Simple picture books
  - Flap and textured books
  - Books with one or two sentences per page
  - Books that rhyme
  - Books with a story that can be discussed

Young children learn so many skills through listening and participating during book reading. Skills such as phonological awareness, vocabulary, sequencing, auditory memory skills will assist with later school success.

For young children, parents can start by looking at simple books with simple visual pictures and provide simple descriptions of the pictures. As children get older and can assist in manipulating the pictures, flap or texture books are great to increase their interest in books. Children also get an idea of the sequence of books by turning pages from the beginning to the end of the book.

- Sing, sing, sing.
  - Songs with hand motions ("Happy and You Know It," "Eensy Weensy Spider," "Hokey Pokey")
  - Songs with refrains ("Farmer in the Dell")
  - Songs with rhymes ("Humpty Dumpty," "Eensy Weensy Spider")

Songs are very calming for very young children. Parents are encouraged to sing as the baby is calming for the night, while in the car, taking a walk, or wherever they are with their child. There are many children's songbooks such as:

  - *The Library of Children's Songs* (Appleby, 1993)
  - *The Fantastic Big Book of Children's Songs* (Leonard, 2004)

○ *101 Music Games for Children* (Storm, 1995)

Several Web sites also provide children's lyrics. These include:

○ KIDiddles (n.d.) (http://www.KIDiddles.com)

○ BusSongs.com (Mander, n.d.) (http://www.bussongs.com)

Singing with their child can continue through early elementary school.

- Talk, talk, talk.
  Parents are encouraged to speak to their child—talk about what is in the room, talk about what the parents are going to do and where they are going. Children will increase vocabulary skills, sequencing, and memory skills by listening and talking to their parents. These are important prerequisite skills for learning.

- Limit television for the child.
  The television provides passive learning and does not allow children to interact. This makes them passive rather than active learners. Children need to experience their environment in order to learn. A parent talking, reading, and singing to their child will provide the opportunity for the child to be an active participant and, thus, learn more about their environment.

- Experience the world through:
  ○ Water play
  ○ Sand play
  ○ Food play
  ○ Yard play
  ○ Trips to children-friendly places (zoo, children's museum, park)

  Parents are encouraged to provide environments and activities that allow their children to develop auditory, tactile, kinesthetic, and visual skills. During trips to familiar places, parents can begin to point out familiar signs (stop sign, name of their bank, restaurants with distinct signs). This will encourage vocabulary development, concept development, category knowledge, and environmental reading, which are an important preliteracy skills and a great step to understanding that whole words have meaning.

In conclusion, regardless of a child's age, the stage is set early for the importance of learning. Parents are the first teachers with a big job to do. Reading, singing, playing, and exploring provides opportunities for receptive and expressive vocabulary and language building, concept development, understanding rhyming, sequencing, understanding events in the past, and, overall, making learning fun.

Home Strategies for Literacy Skills Introduction

I was assisting a second-grade student with math homework (language is everywhere!!) where he had to estimate certain items then provide the actual amount. The first estimation was dishes in one cabinet. Because this child has frequent discrimination errors,

I never take for granted understanding of any words. I asked this student if he knew what a cabinet is. His response was, "Yes." I asked him to explain. He stated that it was a house made of wood. He is thinking that this assignment is silly because how is he going to count plates in a "cabin" when he does not have a cabin! This is an example of a student who continues to struggle with the ability to discriminate words.

Here's How Parents Can Work With Their Student on Developing Literacy Skills

- Practice the visual phonics letter and sounds daily.
  A visual phonics program is presented in chapter 3, Getting Started: Preliteracy Skills. Once this is introduced to the student and the parent in the classroom or in therapy, parents can go through it daily. This will increase phoneme awareness of the alphabet sounds, diagraphs (sh, ch, th, wh), and diphthongs (oi, oy, ow, ou, au, aw).

- Use visual phonics cues to assist the student when perceptual errors occur.
  Parents and teachers should monitor a student's response to directions or when it is obvious that the child did not correctly perceive information presented. For example, I had a little girl ask her mom for "old fish" at the grocery store. The little girl finally took her mom to the snack isle for Gold Fish crackers. I had a little boy look at his mom very perplexed when she was talking about dragging the laundry basket. The little boy perceived "dragon" for "dragging," He was looking for a dragon in the laundry basket. Parents can use the gestures from the visual phonics program to cue their student when a misperception occurs in words.

- Use the visual phonics cues as described in chapter 3 to assist the student with spelling.
  Instead of parents telling their student how to spell a word, they can use the visual phonics cues for that sound so that the student can process the information and spell the word. This is particularly helpful for students with vowel discrimination errors.

- Make sure the student understands all meanings of spelling and vocabulary words.
  This will accomplish several goals: it assists the parent in making sure that the student has perceived these words correctly previously and it increases the student's vocabulary skills.

- Play same or different.
  Parents can play a game of same or different where they provide two words—the same word, a rhyming word, or a word that is perceptual similar (horse and house), and the student has to tell the parent whether the words are the same words or different words. If the student remarks that it is the same word when it is actually a rhyming word, the parent should probe further to assess what the student heard. The parent can then use the visual phonics gesture to provide both words again. The student should listen and watch the visual gestures, then decide if the words are the same or different on the second attempt.

In conclusion, the ability to perceive sounds and words correctly is vital for academic success. One must be able to accurately discriminate one word from another in order to follow directions correctly, to understand a book being read, to follow the teacher's information in the classroom, to write down the correct homework assignment when given verbally, and to understand multiple meanings of words for future learning.

Home Strategies to Increase Auditory Short-Term Memory and Comprehension Introduction

The ability to hold auditory information in short-term memory long enough to repeat a list of items, numbers, a sentence verbatim, or to follow an auditory direction or a classroom lecture is necessary in order to comprehend auditory information and be academically successful. Parents can encourage greater auditory memory skills to lead to great academic success.

- Provide directions of increasing length and complexity for the student to follow.
  - Simple familiar directions (Hands up.)
  - Simple unfamiliar or novel directions (Go to the door.)
  - Two-step related directions (Go to the door, and get your shoes.)
  - Two-step related directions with two or more attributes (Go to the door, and get your new blue shoes.)
  - Directions with a series of items (Get your shoes, backpack, coat, and umbrella.)
  - Two-step unrelated directions (Go to the living room, and get the book on the table.)
  - Two or greater number of steps with time order (First, go to the living room and get the book on the table. Then go upstairs and give it to your sister.)

For a preschool child, the earliest glimpse into auditory short-term memory is a child's ability to follow simple directions (Hands up. Get your shoes). As soon as the child demonstrates success with simple directions, parents can increase the length and complexity of the directions, which would require the child to hold a greater amount of information into auditory memory.

- Have the child repeat sentences while reading a book.
  As a parent is reading a book, he or she can read a page then ask the child to repeat the sentence that was just read.
- Ask the child to retell the story without looking at the book.
  Retelling a story without looking at the book relies on significant auditory memory skills and subsequent comprehension of the story. The parents may want to start by reading a few pages and asking the child to retell that portion of the story. As the child is able to hold greater amount of information into auditory

memory, the parents can increase the number of pages read before asking the child to retell the story.

- Provide a list of items for the student to recall.
  The parents can provide a list of items needed from the store and ask their student to remember a certain amount of items. The amount can increase as the student is successful. If it is a list of items to purchase from a well-known store, the parents can organize the items requested as the student would find them in the store. For example, if the personal item section is first, then toys, then crafts, and finally food, the parent can say, "Please, help me remember to get toothpaste, a toy for Johnny's birthday, paint, and ice cream." This way the student can visualize walking through the store in order and getting those items.

- Play word games to assist with auditory short-term memory.
  As stated in chapter 4, games such as going through each letter of the alphabet and making up a story are a fun way to increase auditory recall. The student has to go through what the others have said then add new information and continue the story. For example, for the letter A, My name is Annie. I am from Alaska, and my brother is Adam. We sell apples. The next person repeats this then adds a story for the letter B.

Home Strategies for Reading Comprehension Introduction

Concentrating on smaller chunks of information that a student is required to read assists him or her to increase comprehension of the information. So instead of starting a chapter in Science such as one on space and reading each section as assigned, the student should read subsection by subsection and grasp the meaning before moving on to the next subsection. The comprehension and recall will be significantly increased. If the student takes notes while reviewing each subsection, comprehension and recall will be further enhanced. Any time the student has time to work ahead and prelearn information for the next day's class, understanding and retaining the information will be greater. An added bonus to taking notes on each subsection will be that the student has all notes needed to study for a test, thus decreasing the time to get study material organized and reviewing to prepare for a test. This means more time to study and better performance on the test.

Here's How to Work on Reading Comprehension at Home

- Students can assist their parents with cooking from a recipe.
  My favorite sugar cookie recipe comes from a *Sesame Street* book (Bove et al., 1983) that I got as part of a series when my children were young. It has pictures to demonstrate ingredients and tools needed as well as a picture for each step to make the cookies. My children would read and measure each ingredient. I continue to use this sugar cook recipe today. Children's cookbooks are

available at any bookstore or online. Parents should find one with pictures of the ingredients and tools needed as well as pictures assisting their student with each step. The student can read each step and use the picture to assist with comprehension. The parent should take the student's lead regarding how to make the dish.

- Do craft activities together.
  I have found that students are more willing to attempt to read while working on a craft. Craft activities can be purchased as a kit from a store or parents can look up a specific craft online or in a book. Again, pictures should be present for the items needed and each step in making the craft. The student should lead the craft, telling the adult what the next step is.

Many children are reluctant readers because it is difficult. If it can be accomplished through a fun activity such as cooking or a craft, the student often is more willing to attempt the reading while working on comprehension at the same time.

- During reading assignments for school, such as Social Studies, Science, and any other areas that require a significant amount of reading, assist the student in following the below format:
  1. **K** What I know
  2. **W** What I want to know
  3. **L** What I learned

  This will provide a framework for what will be in that section. I have found that it is easier for students to change the subsection title into a question in order to discuss what was learned. For example, if the subsection title in Science is "Limestone Rock," they can turn that into a question such as "What is limestone rock" or "Where is limestone rock found?" If the student can answer the question based on what was read, then he or she is ready to take notes on that section and move on to the next session.

- Assist the students with taking notes for increased comprehension.
  As presented in chapter 6, students can use webs or Cornell Notes to take notes on the information learned. Another possibility is to print the chapter information if the publisher provides the textbooks online or copy the pages so that the students can highlight important words while reading.

- Increase reading comprehension for literature.
  One of my "ah ha" moments came while I was working with a student with his summer reading books that were assigned to be read before the beginning of the next school year. This eighth-grade student was listening to the book assigned on MP3 download then was meeting with me to review the information. This is a young man who has struggled with reading fluency, accuracy, and comprehension. After completing this book, he asked me to check online to see if the next book in the series was available and if it was available for download. I checked and sure enough it was. He asked his mom, on that day, to go to the

library as they left my office to get the book. A couple of months later, he was completing a school assignment for history. The assignment asked the student to determine if someone was writing about him what that person would write. The next questions were regarding what he would want the person to write about him that the person may not already know. His response, as an eighth grader, was that he read his first book that year. Reading should be fun—not torture—as it was for this student.

Many books that are assigned for reading in school are available for MP3 download. Students should check with the school librarian to determine if the library will download and loan out an MP3 player or provide on a CD. If it is not available for download through the school library, parents can check with the local library. There also are many Internet sites where parents or students can download books. Parents should encourage their student to read along while listening. Another strategy for reading comprehension of literacy, as presented in chapter 6, is that students can use a book report format to determine the parts of the story. As stated in that chapter, students should be encouraged to read the book summary presented on the back cover of the book. This provides information regarding characters, plot, and setting. From there, the student can make predictions about what the story will be about.

In conclusion, reading comprehension is critical for academic success but often is torture for the students we are so fortunate to have in our lives. If a student is unable to understand the gestalt and the important details, the content will have little meaning. If the content has little meaning, retaining the information will be difficult. If retaining the information is difficult, then success in the classroom and test taking will be adversely affected.

Home Strategies for Critical Thinking Introduction

As discussed previously, from third grade on, students are reading to learn. Along with reading to learn, critical thinking becomes vitally important to make inferences and predictions about information that is being learned. Critical thinking also is necessary in order to link newly learned information to what is already known. Specific subjects also begin to have critical reasoning questions in the section reviews and chapter reviews.

Here's How to Work on Critical Thinking at Home

- Play games to encourage critical thinking.
  Games that require students to make a quick response or ask logical questions are a fun way to work on critical thinking skills. Games such as Guess Who (Milton Bradley, 1982), Guess Where (Milton Bradley, 2004), Crossword puzzles, 10 questions, Clue Great Museum Caper (Hasbro, 1991), Clue Junior: The Case of the Missing Cake (Hasbro, 2003), Outburst (Parker Brothers, 1995), Taboo (Hasbro,

1989), Taboo Junior (Hasbro, 2001), Catch Phrase (Parker Brothers, 1994), and Catch Phrase Junior (Parker Brothers, 2002) are great games for critical thinking.

- Encourage them to attempt the critical thinking items in the Science and Social Studies chapter review even if it is not assigned. For compare or contrast questions, students should make a chart: Compare = how are they the same; Contrast = how are they different.

Compare or Contrast

1st Subject	2nd Subject

Students also can be encouraged to use a Venn diagram as discussed in chapter 6 for concepts that they are asked to compare and contrast. A T chart for comparing or contrasting or a Venn diagram for comparing and contrasting should be used consistently.

In conclusion, critical thinking is necessary for academic success as well as life success. Many decisions are based on the ability to think "What would happen if?" For students without strong critical thinking skills, they will be more apt to go along with someone else's suggestion, which may not always be the best choice. Parents should be encouraged to be consistent with the strategies (T chart and Venn diagrams) or any other strategies used for critical thinking for subject-based information so that their student makes a habit of using the tools for academic success.

Written Expression Introduction

In order to be successful with written expression, students must be able to correctly retrieve words that they know and be able to spell (phonics) the words not known. They must formulate thoughts regarding what to write, organize the information, and then write. Students with retrieval difficulties will often write short, choppy sentences and reduced content. Students with receptive and expressive language disorder and motor planning will demonstrate a decrease in vocabulary usage due to the limitations of their comprehension and use of vocabulary. They also will demonstrate difficulties with content as well as using figurative language (similes, metaphors, expressions, etc.) in order to write an in-depth paper.

Here's How Parents Can Assist Their Student With Written Expression

- Use the following strategy for written expression:
  - Choose a topic, if applicable.
  - Research the topic.

- ○ Generate a list of words that pertain to that topic.
- ○ Place into categories the items from the list.

EXAMPLE: Basketball

1	court	3	uniforms
1	ball	3	shoes
1	backboard	3	mouth guard
1	net	2	scoring
2	2 points	2	3 points
2	Free throws		

The information can then be used to establish a web to organize the information for writing a paragraph or a paper.

- Assist the student with consistently using webs to organize ideas.
  See chapter 5, Across the Curriculum, for the setup of webs. As stated in chapter 5, the main idea goes in a bubble in the middle of the paper. Details go in separate bubbles, starting in the upper left corner and moving clockwise.

- Assist the student with writing complete sentences.
  Each bubble from the web becomes at least one complete sentence. The first sentence is from the middle bubble, which is the main idea. Each detail becomes at least one complete sentence. The last bubble should represent the conclusion. For a paper, the bubbles are the main idea and detail of each paragraph. Usually the information writing in the bubble for the main idea is the thesis statement or the last sentence in the introductory paragraph that explains the content of the paper.

Home Strategies for the Concepts and Language of Math Introduction

I had a parent say recently, "Why does everything, including math, have to involve language?" Math is not just about knowing addition, subtraction, and multiplication math facts or being able to solve math problems. Math is full of vocabulary, concepts, critical thinking, and application. I have students who perform well on math facts timed tests that are prevalent in our schools in first through third grades. Once those math facts have to be used to solve a math story problem or an algebraic expression, the students have significant difficulty.

Here's How to Work on Math at Home

- Encourage the students to use graph paper to solve math problems.
  Graph paper is a great way to keep columns of numbers organized. Graph paper in various sizes can be obtained from Web sites like http://www.dotolearn.com

(n.d.) under Math Helpers. The variety of sizes works well based on the students' fine motor skill.

- Assist the students with using a place value chart for learning whole numbers, decimals, fractions, and rounding.
  A place value chart provides a great visual strategy to assist students with understanding ones, tens, hundreds, thousands, and so on. As discussed many times in this book, new learning should always be based on what the students already know. If the students understand the place value chart, the parents can use this same chart when rounding is introduced.
  It also can be used to explain decimals and fractions.

- Assist the students with using consistent steps for following math story problems. Talk about language and critical thinking in math! Math story problems are really critical thinking with numbers. A concise and consistent method to solving these problems will make understanding these math problems much easier for students. Many math books provide a method for solving story problems. Parents can make this into a chart or copy the page so that it can be used each time story problems are presented. Soon, their student will internalize the process and will be able to use it without the visual reminder. Following is a method that can be used. This strategy is based on the strategy for following written directions where students underline the important words before trying to complete the assignment.
  - Read the problem carefully.
  - Read the problem again.
    - Underline important words.
    - The sentence that begins with "What" tells you what you need to solve.
  - Look for key words that also should be underlined
  - Associate numbers with important information and write down that information.
    - For example: A piece of property valued at $55,000 (property value = 55,000)
  - Identify a starting point based on what the question is asking.
  - Solve the problem.
  - Reread to make sure you answered the question that is being asked.

- Assist students with understanding the vocabulary and concepts of math.
  The folded vocabulary cards described previously and presented in chapter 5 work well for both new math vocabulary and concepts. For both vocabulary and concepts, the folded card should be used as described in chapter 5. The difference is where a picture to provide the visual representation would be placed for other vocabulary, application examples would be placed in that location for math.

In conclusion, it would be so nice if students with speech and/or language disorders could have one school subject that did not include language. I have yet to find one! Language strategies can apply to math concepts for the students' success with the language and critical thinking aspects of math.

Conclusion

Parents are the first educators of the students we see. They lay the foundation for their child's ongoing learning experiences. By providing parents the tools to continue this education of their children, we will have a cohesive team to assist student learning. From the development of preliteracy skills to assisting with learning strategies, parents play a vital role in their child's education.

References

Appleby, A. (1993). *The library of children's song classics* (Bk ed.). New York, NY: Music Sales America.

Bove, L., Frith, M., Kingsley, E. P., Learner, S., Moss, J., Stiles, N., et al. (1983). *The Sesame Street treasure volume 1*. New York, NY: Random House. (Out of print)

Do to Learn. (n.d.). Math Helpers [Computer program]. Retrieved October 1, 2009, from http://www.dotolearn.com

Hasbro. (1991). Clue Great Museum Caper. Pawtucket, RI: Author.

Hasbro. (2003). Clue Junior: The Case of the Missing Cake. Pawtucket, RI: Author.

Hasbro. (1998). Taboo. Pawtucket, RI: Author.

Hasbro. (2001). Taboo Junior. Pawtucket, RI: Author.

KIDiddles. (n.d.). "The Bee." Retrieved February 22, 2009, from http://www.kididdles.com/lyrics/b048.html

Leonard, H. (2004). *The fantastic big book of children's songs*. New York, NY: Hal Leonard.

Mander, K. (n.d.). Children's Songs & Nursery Rhymes with Lyrics, Words & Music. Retrieved November 7, 2009, from http://www.bussongs.com

Milton Bradley. (2004). Guess Where. Pawtucket, RI: Author.

Milton Bradley. (1992). Guess Who. Pawtucket, RI: Author.

Parker Brothers. (1994). Catch Phrase. Pawtucket, RI: Author.

Parker Brothers. (2002). Catch Phrase Junior. Pawtucket, RI: Author.

Parker Brothers. (1995). Outburst. Pawtucket, RI: Author.

Storm, J. (1995). *101 Music games for children: Fun and learning with rhythm and song (SmartFun Activity Books)*. Alameda, CA: Hunter House.

10

The Greatest Resources

Introduction

So many great resources are available through books, workbooks, Internet sites, and applications (apps) based devices such as smart phones or tablet devices. The wealth of information is sometimes overwhelming with new information available almost daily. It is amazing how many free Web sites are available that provide materials for educators, speech-language pathologists, and parents.

Evidence-based practice calls for us to know the research, use our clinical judgment and expertise, as well as consider the family/student perspective. Some of the materials listed may not have a significant research base but are well marketed to professionals and families.

As professionals we need to be aware of these resources. Speech-language pathologists are encouraged to compare research and other information provided on the American Speech-Language-Hearing Association (ASHA) Web site (http://www.asha.org) with other resources regarding specific topics.

This chapter provides categories of information that have been discussed throughout this text. It provides resources for supporting material that can be used to work with students who need assistance in specific areas. It also offers a brief description of what the resources offer.

Childhood Apraxia of Speech (CAS)

CAS with a comorbid language disorder can significantly impact academic success. A significant knowledge base regarding the disorder and appropriate intervention strategies can decrease the academic struggles for these students.

Here's How to Treat Childhood Apraxia of Speech

The first part of this book defines and describes characteristics of CAS. A protocol for an effective treatment is described, including phoneme sequencing, repetitive practice, intensity of treatment, selection of vocabulary, and use of multisensory cues to facilitate improvement of motor speech skills. Additional considerations such as vowel production, prosody, and production of phrases and sentences are included. The book also includes resources for parents (Fish, 2010).

American Speech-Language-Hearing Association (ASHA)

ASHA (n.d.) offers many resources regarding CAS. These include its position statement, research, and presentations.

Kaufman Children's Center

Nancy Kaufman, Speech-Language Pathologist, is the director of Kaufman Children's Center for Speech, Language, Sensory Motor, and Social Connections. The center offers information on the early signs and symptoms of apraxia of speech as well as other speech diagnoses (Kaufman, n.d.).

The Late Talker: What to Do If Your Child Isn't Talking Yet

This book was introduced to me by several parents of the students I see. There is little evidence-based information in this book. However, it provides some basic information for parents as they begin to explore CAS and comorbid language difficulties. This book includes a chapter on nutritional support that discusses the use of omega 3 fatty acids (Agin, Geng, & Nicholl, 2004).

Apraxia-KIDS

Apraxia-KIDS is a program of the Childhood Apraxia of Speech Association. Its Web site (http://www.apraxia-kids.org) offers information regarding verbal apraxia for parents and professionals (Apraxia-KIDS, n.d.). It includes an overall description of CAS. Diagnosis and treatment information is also provided as well as a family start guide with general information about CAS. Apraxia-KIDS sponsors an annual conference regarding CAS.

Word Finding

A word-finding disorder is an expressive disorder affecting single word, discourse, and oral reading. It can impact a student retrieving basic concepts such as colors and shapes to the recall of alphabet letter names, sounds of letters, sight words, and use of vocabulary. Students with word-finding difficulties also demonstrate difficulty with oral reading and written expression.

American Speech-Language-Hearing Association (ASHA)

ASHA offers many resources regarding word finding. This includes research and presentations offered at the national conventions.

Word-Finding Difficulties

The Word Finding Web site (http://www.wordfinding.com) provides information about word finding for professionals, parents, and those with word-finding difficulties. Topics presented include definition and characteristics, word-finding assessment and intervention, and available course work (German, n.d.).

The book *It's on the Tip of My Tongue* (German, 2001) discusses word-finding strategies to remember names and words.

Word Finding Intervention Program 2 (WFIP 2)

WFIP 2 (German, 2005) offers a comprehension intervention program that focuses on three areas:

- Retrieval Strategy Instruction
- Self-Advocacy Instruction
- Word-Finding Accommodations

Dual-Focus Vocabulary Instruction for Word Finding, Meanings, and Retrieval Strategies, a presentation offered at ASHA's national convention, provides strategies to target storage and retrieval strength for vocabulary to assist those with word-finding difficulties (German, 2007).

The Brain and Language

A basic understanding of the brain's function is a necessity for all who are working with students with learning differences. By being able to take what one observes diagnostically and linking it to brain function, other characteristics seen in these students begin to make greater sense. For example, if a student has attention and impulsivity issues coupled with difficulty with social skills and problem solving, it is more than likely that the student has prefrontal lobe dysfunction. By understanding this, the treatment plan should reflect more than working on reasoning skills—it also should address how working on reasoning skills and understanding the gestalt and details that support the main idea will lead to great social skills.

Executive Skills in Children and Adolescents: A Practical Guide to Assessment and Intervention (Practical Intervention in the Schools)

This book is an excellent resource manual that provides a research-based framework for strengthening executive functioning in children and adolescents. The book explains how executive skills develop in children and are used in everyday life (Dawson & Guare, 2010).

BrainGym.com

This Web site provides sources for physical movement patterns to assist in learning. Paul Dennison (n.d.) describes human brain function in terms of three dimensions: laterality, focus, and centering. Laterality is the crossover between both sides of the brain. Laterality skills are fundamental to reading, writing, listening, or speaking. Focus dimension is the connection of the back and front areas of the brain. This dimension is to increase comprehension. The centering dimension is the connection between the top and bottom structures of the brain. Centering enables us to harmonize emotion with rational thought. The purpose of Brain Gym exercises is centered around these three dimensions, and benefits include improvements in learning, vision, memory, expression, and movement abilities.

Brain-Based Learning: The New Science of Teaching and Training

This text provides foundational information for understanding brain-based teaching techniques that can dramatically improve student performance and success in the classroom (Jensen, 2000).

How the Brain Learns to Read

This book provides the most current neuroscientific information regarding reading and effective learning for reading success (Sousa, 2004).

How the Brain Learns

This book provides some of the most research on brain functioning and translates this information into effective classroom strategies and activities (Sousa, 2006).

How the Special Needs Brain Learns

This book provides an overview of a variety of special learning needs accompanied by practical information about how to address those needs. It makes understanding the relationship between the special learning need and the brain easier to understand (Sousa, 2007).

The Leadership Brain: How to Lead Today's Schools More Effectively

This book provides information regarding brain-compatible leadership practices that sustain effective school leadership, team management, teaching, and learning. It includes understanding the differences in learning and retention, left and right hemispheric preferences, and higher-order thinking. It also provides misconceptions about students with disabilities, those who are gifted, and minority students (Sousa, 2003).

Developmental Language Disorders

This text provides current knowledge regarding neurological development, neuroimaging techniques, and research on the neurological basis of language disorders, autism, reading (dyslexia), and genetic conditions (Williams, 2008).

Literacy

Literacy is the basis of learning. One needs to be able to read fluently and comprehend what is read in order to understand all academic areas and to be successful academically. We, as educators, should understand what we are seeing in young children regarding the indicators of literacy success (i.e., preliteracy skills of phonological awareness, narrative skills, short-term auditory memory, and sequencing). We also need to have open eyes regarding red flags that indicate that a child may demonstrate literacy difficulties due to difficulties with preliteracy skills. School is a student's work. The student must be successful in his or her work. Literacy is the foundation of success.

American Speech-Language-Hearing Association (ASHA)

ASHA offers many resources regarding literacy development in addition to research regarding speech and language disorders and comorbid learning disabilities. These include its position statement, research, and presentations offered at its national conventions.

Carl's Corner

This free Web site (http://carlscorner.us.com) offers a plethora of resources for literacy. For example, it offers many activities for high-frequency words, word families, nursery rhymes, contractions, holiday, reading fluency, plus many, many more (Carl's Corner, n.d.).

abcteach.com

This site provides free worksheets in addition to other resources for members. It provides worksheets and printable pages for reading comprehension, flashcards, themes, research and reports, and many other areas (abcteach, n.d.).

Sing Me a Story

This book provides several popular children's stories. It provides song lyrics to tell the story and also includes ideas for vocabulary, picture symbols, and several language activities (Maida, 2010).

National Institute for Literacy (NIFL)

The NIFL (n.d.), a federal agency, provides leadership on literacy issues, including the improvement of reading instruction for children, youth, and adults. *Put Reading First: Kindergarten through Grade 3* is a resource that is offered on the NIFL Web site. It has three sections regarding children and students: early intervention, childhood, and adolescence. Each section includes key literacy issues, reading components, teaching approaches, and research (Armbruster, Osborne, & Lehr, 2001).

Road to Reading: A Program for Preventing and Remediating Reading Difficulties

This book provides a step-by-step program for struggling readers. *Road to Reading* is designed for educators of students in the first through third grades but also can be used with older students who still struggle with reading. The program addresses sound-symbol correspondences, decoding skills, phonetically regular words, high-frequency words, oral reading in context, and dictation (Blachman & Tangel, 2008).

ClickN READ Phonics®

The clicknkids (n.d.) Web site (http://www.clicknkids.com) provides two excellent researched-based phonics and high-frequency word programs. ClickN READ is a research-based Internet program that includes letter/sound identification; keyboard spelling for letter sounds; word blending; identification of sounds in the beginning, middle, and end of words; word and sentence reading; sight word reading; word families; affixes; and story reading. This same Web site also offers ClickN SPELL, a research-based spelling program for prekindergarten through fifth grade that teaches the 800 most commonly used words in the English language.

Earobics

This research-based program builds students' skills in phonemic awareness, auditory processing, and phonics as well as the cognitive and language skills required for comprehension. Each level of instruction addresses recognizing and blending sounds, rhyming, and discriminating phonemes within words and adjusts to each student's ability level (Earobics, n.d.).

HearBuilder's Phonological Awareness

This program is designed to target nine phonological processes. These include phoneme, syllable and sentence segmentation, phoneme and syllable blending, rhyming, phoneme identification, phoneme deletion, addition, and manipulation (HearBuilder, n.d.).

Discover Lexercise

Lexercise is a Web-based program built on Orton Gillingham principles. It targets morphology, phonology, syllable types, and phoneme-grapheme pairs for literacy development (Myers & Blackley, n.d.).

Hubbard's Cupboard

This free Web site offers information for prekindergarten curriculum (Hubbard's Cupboard, n.d.). It also offers a literacy section that includes guided and shared reading, rhymes, printable books (sight word and word family books), sight words, and story lessons (e.g., Literacy).

Reading Rockets

This Web site offers a variety of reading strategies, lessons, and activities designed to help young children and struggling readers learn how to read and improve their reading skills (Meier, n.d.).

Kidzone

This Web site offers activities, such as Preschool Printing Practice, based on age/grade level and subject areas. This includes activities for math, reading, science, and geography (Kidzone, n.d.).

Phonics

This program offers phonics and spelling programs based on an Orton-Gillingham approach. VoWac (n.d.) provides instruction in word decoding and spelling strategies.

Reading A-Z

This Web site offers thousands of downloadable materials for assessment, guided reading, phonemic awareness, reading comprehension, reading fluency, alphabet, and vocabulary (Reading A-Z, n.d.).

ReadWriteThink

This Web site offers student materials divided into three main sections: learning language, learning about language, learning through language. Learning language includes using language in everyday activities. Learning about language includes letter/sound relationships, spelling, and grammar. Learning through language includes using reading and writing to learn subject-based material (n.d.).

PreLiteracy.com

This free Web site offers hand cues for a multisensory approach to teaching letters and letter sounds.

Written Language Expression

Written language is the culmination of all language areas joined together with visual motor skills. It includes the ability to express oneself in a format that relies on spelling, sentence formulation, paragraph formulation, thought organization, visual motor skills, and fine motor skills.

Step Up to Writing

Step Up to Writing (Auman, 1999) is a program that is used often in the classroom for expository writing (inform, explain, describe, or define the subject). It teaches writing strategies within the writing process (prewriting, drafting, revising, editing, final copy, proofreading, sharing) to help students organize their thinking and writing. Each element of expository writing (thesis statement, topic sentences, transitions, examples, and conclusion) is color coded in the organization phase.

The Writing Lab Approach to Language Instruction

The Writing Lab Approach to Language Instruction (Wolf Nelson, Barh, & Van Meter, 2004) provides computer-supported activities that focus on the five language domains (morphology, phonology, semantics, syntax, and pragmatics).

The Story Grammar Marker

The Story Grammar Marker (Moreau & Fidrych, 1994) uses manipulative tools and resources that help students in Grades 2 through 6 develop reading, writing, and speaking skills.

Draft Builder

This program provides a means for brainstorming, note taking, and writing drafts (Don Johnston Incorporated, n.d.).

Writing Tools

This section of the Web site provides different styles of writing paper for beginning hand-writing skills (Do to Learn, n.d.).

Inspiration Software, Inc.

This software company provides visual organizational strategies through two programs. Kidspiration for students in kindergarten through Grade 5 and Inspiration for those in Grades 6 through 12. These programs use idea maps to stimulate ideas about a topic, concept maps to link information together, and webs for organization and prewriting.

Math

Would it not be wonderful if a student who struggles with speech and language, language processing, retrieval, reading, and reading comprehension could have one academic area or an area of life that did not include language? For many students, math computation comes easily, but the application of the math is difficult. Math story problems rely on language/reading comprehension and reasoning skills before the computation can begin. Students must figure out what the problem is then figure out how to solve it.

TouchMath

This learning tool is a multisensory program that uses corresponding points on the numbers. It provides a step-by-step approach for counting, addition, subtraction, place value, multiplication, division, time, money, fractions, story problems, shapes, sizes, and pre-algebra (Innovative Learning Concepts, n.d.).

Math Helpers

Do to Learn (n.d.) is a Web site that offers free assistance in many areas. Math Helpers is located under the Activities icon at the top of the homepage. This section provides grid paper of various sizes, 100s chart for addition and subtraction, a multiplication table, and a vertical number line.

Classroom Organizers/Schedules

Classroom organizers/schedules provide a visual representation to assist students with organization in the classroom. This can be from using pictures to label centers for the younger children to schedule boards to assist with knowing what will come next in the day to assisting with transitions from subject to subject. For the younger children, the daily schedule with pictures can be sent home so that the students can tell others about their school day. Many students with language-based learning disabilities have difficulty with sequencing. The pictures provide the students with a graphic representation of the day's events and aids in the sequencing and recall of events that occurred.

Make a Schedule

The Do to Learn (n.d.) Web site provides many free tools for working with students with special learning needs. This includes calendars and take-home folders. The Make a Schedule program must be purchased on this site. It provides over 2,500 pictures that can be printed in color and black and white. The printed word associated with the picture can be translated into English, Spanish, German, French, Dutch, and Portuguese.

Board Maker

The Mayer-Johnson (n.d.) Web site offers a program for making picture systems. It offers Board Maker Plus, a program that can be used to make schedule boards, calendars, or pictures to organize the classroom. It also offers voice, sound, animation, and video capability.

Images/Sounds and Pictures

In addition to the programs discussed previously, classroom organizers and schedules can be made by making a table using the computer then using Google Images or symbols/pictures from the computer that are available through the "Insert symbol."

Graphic Organizers

Using graphic organizers provides a consistent learning strategy for students. An environment that uses consistent visual strategies provides students with an avenue to visually process through information for increased organization.

Cause and Effect Graphic Organizers

Education Oasis (n.d.) is a free Web site that provides several visual organizers such as Cause and Effect graphic organizers that can be used to figure out what caused an event and the possible consequences of the event. These include herringbone charts, webs, and T charts.

Freeology.com

The Freeology.com (n.d.) Web site provides over 60 graphic organizers that can be printed for free. The organizers include the following:

- Venn Diagrams
  - Double Venn Diagram for comparing/contrasting two topics

- Triple Venn Diagram for comparing/contrasting three topics
- Column Venn Diagram with the similarities column in the middle and the contrasting columns on each side
- Cornell Notes
- Web
- Visual Strategies for Story Comprehension
  - Characterization analyzes five ways to view a character
  - Analyzing short stories
  - Fishbone to organize thoughts about a story based on the who, what, where, when, and why
  - Reading response chart
  - Prereading chart
  - SQ3R for Survey, Question, Read, Retell, and Review
  - KWL for what the students know, what they want to know, and what they learn

Inspiration Software, Inc.

This Web site provides graphic organizers for students from kindergarten through high school through two programs. The program for the younger students is Kidspiration with Inspiration being for the older students. The two programs offer the following:

- Kidspiration is designed for students from kindergarten to Grade 5. It provides concept mapping for organization of thoughts and information. It allows students to add pictures and text to explain the main idea and details. It also has a section that provides visual graphics for the students to learn basic math skills such as counting, place value, and geometric understanding.
- Inspiration is designed for students from Grades 6 through 12. It allows students to organize information using a web format or an outline format then toggle between the two. Whatever the students add in either format is added to the other format as well. The students can add pictures and text for greater understanding. Hyperlinks as well as videos can be added.

Using Visual Maps

The Do to Learn (n.d.) Web site has many free materials as well as materials that require membership (e.g., schedule maker). The visual map section of this Web site provides free graphic organizers. The following organizers are available:

- Brainstorming Map: The key concept is placed in the middle largest circle. Elements are placed on either side of the key concept with details in circles below each element.

- Concept Map: This map provides a way to graphically link key concepts, definitions, details, and examples.
- Data Chart: This chart is used to list observations in order to provide a visual representation of the information.
- Decision-Making Guide: This guide provides an excellent visual way to list issues, options, and pros/cons of the decisions that may be made from choosing a specific option. This is a great organizer for students who have to do a persuasive speech or paper.
- Hierarchical Organizer: This organizer lists the topic, subtopics, and details with the topic at the top of the page, subtopics under the topic, and details under the subtopics.
- T Chart: The T chart is a great way to compare or contrast topics.

Study Skills and Test-Taking Strategies

Consistent strategies for learning material through test taking can assist students with any learning disability have an organized way to attack the areas that affect knowledge and performance.

Study Skills

This workbook provides 46 exercises including scheduling, outlining, note-taking, memorizing, test-taking (essay and objective), and reference tools. This workbook is designed for students in Grades 5 through 8 (Remedia Publications, 1998).

Test-Taking Strategies

This workbook offers activities focused on listening for directions, following directions, skimming and scanning, test-taking terminology, the process of elimination, using word clues, recognizing question stems, and using a bubble sheet (Remedia Publications, 1998).

E-Z Test Readiness (Study Skills)

These grade level workbooks prepare students for taking standardized tests (Weiler, 2000).

Classroom Amplification

The Lightspeed Web site provides products for classroom audio systems. It also provides research information regarding classroom performance when a classroom audio system is used with all students.

The Laws

In order to be the best advocate for those we serve, we need to understand the laws that are established so that all students receive an appropriate education. This section provides the federal Web sites that oversee how each state interprets these laws and each state's approach with reaching compliancy with the laws. Speech-language pathologists and all educators also need to look at their state educational laws in order to be the best advocate for each student we proudly serve.

Americans with Disabilities Act (ADA)

The ADA Web site, sponsored by the federal government, provides overall information regarding the ADA. It includes federal resources, publications, and state and local regulations (ADA, n.d.).

Individuals with Disabilities Education Act (IDEA)

The Individuals with Disabilities Education Act (IDEA) is a law ensuring services to children with disabilities throughout the nation from early intervention through high school (up to 21st birthday). Information regarding this law is provided by the U.S. Department of Education through its Web site at http://idea.ed.gov (IDEA, n.d.).

U.S. Department of Education Home Page

This federal government Web site provides information for students, parents, educators, and administrators regarding how to promote student achievement and preparation for global competitiveness by fostering educational excellence and ensuring equal access for all students to educational opportunities (U.S. Department of Education, n.d.).

General Information

Many independent Web sites support educational efforts. These Web sites offer educators and parents resources in order to better understand the students for whom we work as well as a resource of services that these students are entitled to.

LD OnLine

This Web site covers learning differences and disabilities. It is a valuable resource for parents and educators working with students with learning difficulties. It also provides guidance regarding attention deficit disorder, dyslexia, dysgraphia, dyscalculia, dysnomia, reading difficulties, and speech/language disorders LD OnLine, n.d.).

National Assessment of Educational Progress (NAEP)

This Web site collects data to measure the success of academic programs in the United States, known as *The Nation's Report Card* (NAEP, n.d.). The National Center for Education Statistics (NCES) is the primary federal entity for collecting and analyzing data related to education.

Conclusion

This is by no means a complete list of the most valuable resources. New resources are available every day. This list is meant to be a starting point of materials that can make our job easier. It also is meant as a resource in order to better understand students with learning differences. Lastly, it is meant as a starting point to understanding the laws that govern the rights of all students. There are many great resources available to us. Our greatest resource is one another and the dialogue and problem solving that we can share. Together, we can have a significant impact on the academic life for those we are so privileged to serve.

References

abcteach. (n.d.). Retrieved February 22, 2011, from http://abcteach.com

Agin, M., Geng, L., & Nicholl, M. (2004). *The late talker: What to do if your child isn't talking yet* (Introduction, p. XVIII). New York, NY: St. Martin's Griffin.

American Speech-Language-Hearing Association (ASHA). (n.d.). Retrieved January 23, 2011, from http://www.asha.org

Americans with Disabilities Act. (n.d.). Retrieved February 18, 2011, from http://www.ada.gov

Armbruster, B., Osborne, J., & Lehr, F. (2001). *Put reading first: Kindergarten through grade 3.* Retrieved February 18, 2011, from http://nifl.gov

Auman, M. (1999). Step Up to Writing (Computer program). Dallas, TX: Cambium Learning, Inc.

Blachman, B. A., & Tangel, D. M. (2008). *Road to reading: A program for preventing and remediating reading difficulties.* Baltimore, MD: Paul H. Brookes.

Carl's Corner. (n.d.) Retrieved February 20, 2011, from http://carlscorner.us.com

Childhood Apraxia of Speech Association. (n.d.).

Apraxia-KIDS. Retrieved February 18, 2011, from http://www.apraxia-kids.org

Clicknkids. (n.d.). ClickN READ Phonics® [Computer program]. Retrieved February 18, 2011, from http://www.clicknkids.com

Dawson, P., & Guare, R. (2010). *Executive skills in children and adolescents: A practical guide to assessment and intervention (practical intervention in the Schools)* (2nd ed.). New York, NY: The Guilford Press.

Dennison, P. (n.d.). BrainGym. Retrieved February 18, 2011, from http://braingym.com

Don Johnston Incorporated. (n.d.). Draft Builder [Computer program]. Retrieved February 18, 2011, from http://www.donjohnston.com

Earobics. (n.d.). Earobics [Computer program]. Retrieved February 18, 2011, from http://www.earobics.com

Education Oasis. (n.d.). Cause and Effect Graphic Organizers. Retrieved February 18, 2011, from http://www.educationoasis.com/

Do to Learn. (n.d.). Make a Schedule [Computer program]. Retrieved February 18, 2011, from http://dotolearn.com

Do to Learn. (n.d.). Math Helpers. Retrieved October 1, 2009, from http://www.dotolearn.com

Do to Learn. (n.d.). Visual Map Organizers. Retrieved February 18, 2011, from http://dotolearn.com

Do to Learn. (n.d.). Writing Tools. Retrieved February 18, 2011, from http://dotolearn.com

Fish, M. (2010). *Here's how to treat childhood apraxia of speech.* San Diego, CA. Plural.

Freeology.com. (n.d.). Free Printable Graphic Organizers. Retrieved February 18, 2011, from http://freeology.com/graphicorgs/index.php

German, D. (n.d.). *Word finding difficulties.* Retrieved February 18, 2011, from http://www.wordfinding.com

German, D. (2005). *Word-finding intervention program* (2nd ed.). Austin, TX: Pro-Ed.

German, D. (2007, January 19). *Dual-focus vocabulary instruction for word finding, meanings, and retrieval strategies.* Lecture conducted from American Speech-Language-Hearing Association National Convention, Boston, MA.

HearBuilder. (n.d.). HearBuilder's Phonological Awareness [Computer program]. Retrieved February 18, 2011 from http://www.hearbuilder.com/phonologicalAwareness/

Hubbard's Cupboard. (n.d.). *Literacy.* Retrieved February 18, 2011, from http://wwww.hubbardscupboard.org

Individuals with Disabilities Education Act (IDEA). (n.d.). *Building the legacy of IDEA 2004.* Retrieved February 18, 2011, from http://idea.ed.gov

Innovative Learning Concepts. (n.d.). TouchMath. Retrieved February 18, 2011, from http://www.touchmath.com

Inspiration Software, Inc. (n.d.). Kidspiration and Inspiration [Computer programs]. Retrieved February 18, 2011, from http://www.inspiration.com

Jensen, E. (2000). *Brain-based learning: The new science of teaching and training* (Rev. Ed.). New York, NY: Brain Store.

Kaufman, N. (n.d.). Kaufman Children's Center. Retrieved January 23, 2011, from http://kidspeech.com

Kidzone. (n.d.). Preschool Printing Practice. Retrieved February 18, 2011, from http://www.kidzone.ws/prek_wrksht/dynamic.htm

LD OnLine. (n.d.). Retrieved February 18, 2011, from http://www.ldonline.org

Lightspeed. (n.d.). Retrieved February 18, 2011, from http://www.lightspeed-tek.com

Maida, L. (2010). *Sing me a story.* Lakewood. Stories Unlimited Publication.

Mayer Johnson. (n.d.). Board Maker [Computer program]. Retrieved February 18, 2011, from http://www.mayer-johnson.com

Meier, J. (n.d.). Reading Rockets: Reading Comprehension & Language Arts Teaching Strategies for Kids. Retrieved February 18, 2011, from http://readingrockets.org

Moreau, M., & Fidrych, H. (1994). The Story Grammar Marker [Computer program]. Springfield, MA. Mindwing Concepts. Inc.

Myers, C., & Barrie Blackley, S. (n.d.). Discover Lexercise [Computer program]. Retrieved February 18, 2011, from http://www.lexercise.com

National Assessment of Educational Progress (NAEP). (n.d.). *The nation's report card.* Retrieved February 18, 2011, from http://nces.ed.gov/nationsreportcard

National Institute for Literacy. (n.d.). Retrieved February 18, 2011, from http://www.nifl.gov/

PreLiteracy.com. (n.d.). Retrieved February 22, 2009, from http://www.preliteracy.com

Reading A-Z. (n.d.). Retrieved February 18, 2011, from http://www.readinga-z.com

ReadWriteThink. (n.d.). Retrieved February 18, 2011, from http://www.readwritethink.org/student_mat/index.asp

Remedia Publications. (1998). *Study skills.* Scottsdale, AZ: Author.

Remedia Publications. (1998). *Test-taking strategies.* Scottsdale, AZ: Author.

Sousa, D. (2003). *The leadership brain: How to lead today's schools more effectively.* Thousand Oaks, CA: Corwin Press.

Sousa, D. (2004). *How the brain learns to read.* Thousand Oaks, CA: Corwin Press.

Sousa, D. (2006). *How the brain learns.* Thousand Oaks, CA: Corwin Press.

Sousa, D. (2007). *How the special needs brain learns.* Thousand Oaks, CA: Corwin Press.

U.S. Department of Education. (n.d.). Retrieved March 8, 2009, from U.S. Department of Education Home Page at http://www.ed.gov/

VoWac Publishing Co. (n.d.). Phonics [Computer program]. Retrieved February 18, 2011, from http://www.vowac.com/

Weiler, E. (2000). *E-Z test readiness (Study skills).* Scottsdale, AZ: Remedia Publications.

Williams, D. L. (2008). *Developmental language disorders.* San Diego, CA: Plural.

Wolf Nelson, N., Barh, C., & Van Meter, A. (2004). *The writing lab approach to language instruction and intervention.* Baltimore, MD: Brookes.

Glossary

Abstract reasoning: The ability to understand information on a complex level through problem solving and understanding of figurative language, idioms, and expressions.

Accommodations: Modifications or adjustments to the school environment or educational requirements that will enable a student with a disability to participate in the academic environment to his or her fullest potential.

Achievement: The academic performance of a student.

Alliteration: Repeated consonant sounds occurring at the beginning of words or within words.

Alphabetic principle: The systematic and predictable relationship between written letters and spoken sounds.

Americans with Disabilities Amendments Act of 2004 (ADAA): The law that amends the Americans with Disabilities Act and has a direct impact on Section 504 of the Rehabilitation Act.

Assistive technology: Any technological devices that can enhance the learning opportunities of a student.

Associative reasoning: The ability to reason based on attempting to make a connection between two thoughts or ideas.

Auditory comprehension: The ability to correctly perceive and understand meaning of information.

Auditory processing disorder (APD): Also known as central auditory processing disorder. An impairment of the ability to locate and lateralize sound; discriminate auditory information, and recognize sound patterns. Difficulty with processing auditory information.

Auditory short-term memory: Short-term memory is the active process of storing and retaining information heard through the auditory channel for a limited time.

Body awareness: The internal sense that tells you where your body parts are without your having to look at them. Body awareness is also referred to as proprioception.

Brain stem: Located in front of the cerebellum and extends down to connect to the spinal column. Neurological functions located in the brain stem include those necessary for survival such as breathing; digestion; heart rate; blood pressure; and for basic attention, arousal, and consciousness.

Childhood Apraxia of Speech (CAS): Defined by the American Speech-Language-Hearing Association (ASHA) as "a neurological childhood (pediatric) speech sound disorder in which the precision and consistency of movements underlying speech are impaired in the absence of neuromuscular deficits. CAS may occur as a result of known neurological impairment, in association with complex neurobehavioral disorders of known or unknown origin, or as an idiopathic neurogenic speech sound disorder. The core impairment in planning and/or programming spatiotemporal parameters of movement sequences results in errors in speech sound production and prosody (ASHA, 2007).

Colloquialisms: Informal use of speech by a particular group or geographical area.

Corpus callosum: Nerve tissue that connects the two cerebral hemispheres, allowing communication between the right and left sides of the brain.

Cultural differences: Differences between groups of people based on beliefs, shared attitudes, values, and practices.

Deductive reasoning: The reasoning that starts from the general rule and moves to specific rules.

Digraph: A pair of letters representing a single sound (e.g., /ph/, /ch/, /sh/, /th/).

Diphthong: Two vowel sounds produced together (e.g., au, aw, oi, ou, ow).

Discrepancy: The significant difference between areas. This could include a significant difference between verbal and nonverbal intelligence scores, intelligence and achievement, receptive and expressive language or vocabulary, or a significant discrepancy between any test scores.

Discrimination: The ability to accurately perceive the differences between individual sounds and sounds in words.

Discourse: The language form and function of spoken and written language.

English proficiency: Competency in speaking and understanding the English language. Lack of English proficiency is NOT a learning disability.

Expressive vocabulary: Vocabulary that one uses to express oneself.

Free appropriate public education (FAPE): A significant cornerstone to the Rehabilitation Act and specifically Section 504 of this act. A child with a disability in the United States cannot be excluded from the participation in, be denied the benefits of, or be subjected to discrimination under any program or activity receiving federal financial assistance solely due to the disability.

Graphic organizers: Visual strategies used to assist the student in organizing, understanding, and remembering important information.

Heredity: A biological process wherein genetic information is passed from one generation to the next.

Hyperbole: An exaggerated statement used to heighten effect. It is not used to mislead the reader, but rather to emphasize a point.

Idioms: Language-specific expressions.

Imagery: Descriptions of people or objects stated in terms of our senses.

Individuals with Disabilities Education Act 2004 (IDEA 2004): The latest reauthorization of IDEA and places further emphasis on a quick response when difficulties are noted with a student. It was reauthorized in 2008.

Inductive reasoning: The reasoning that starts from understanding the specifics and deriving a general rule.

Intellectual capacity: The potential intellectual ability of a person.

KWL: A reading comprehension strategy based on what the student knows, what the student hopes to learn, and what the student learned.

Language-based learning disability: Described by the American Speech-Language-Hearing Association (ASHA) as problems with age-appropriate reading, spelling, and/or writing. This disorder is not about how smart a person is.

Learning disability: Children with a learning disability may have difficulty reading, writing, spelling, reasoning, recalling, and/or organizing information.

Lemma: The abstract form of a word that arises after the word has been selected mentally, but before any information has been accessed about the sounds in it. It contains information about the meaning and the relation of this word to others in the sentence.

Long-term memory: Refers to information that has been stored and that is available over a long period.

Metacognition: The process of developing a plan of action, maintaining, monitoring, and evaluating the plan.

Metalinguistic: Language meaning is greater than the words that are used. The ability to reflect consciously on the nature and properties of language (referents, multiple meaning of words, puns, riddles, humor, etc.).

Metaphor: A figure of speech in which an expression is used to suggest a similarity.

Mitigating measures: Defined under the Americans with Disabilities Act as medications and assistive devices that an individual uses to eliminate or reduce the effects of an impairment. Under the Americans with Disabilities Amendments Act of 2008, mitigating measures can only be considered on a limited basis.

Modifications: Actual changes made to curriculum, assignments, tests, and other academic materials and requirements.

No Child Left Behind Act of 2001 (NCLB): The law that places greater accountability to identify and appropriately educate all students.

Onomatopoeia: The use of words that mimic sounds. They appeal to our sense of hearing and they help bring a description to life.

Onset and rime: In a syllable, the onset is the initial consonant or consonants, and the rime is the vowel and any consonants that follow (e.g., in the word *cat*, the onset is "c" and the rime is "at").

Parentally placed private school student: A situation where parents choose to send their student to a private school regardless of disability or availability of services in the public school.

Personification: A figure of speech that gives the qualities of a person to an animal, an object, or an idea. It is a comparison that the author uses to show something in an entirely new light, to communicate a certain feeling or attitude toward it, and to control the way a reader perceives it.

Phonemic awareness: The ability to hear the individual sounds that make up words and the understanding that words are composed of segments of sounds smaller than syllables.

Phonics: Teaching how to connect the sounds of letters or group of letters (e.g., /c/, /k/, /ck/) and how to blend the sounds of letters together to produce unknown words.

Phonological awareness: Understanding of word sound structure and how it can be broken down into smaller units. It includes segmenting words into syllables, segmenting words into individual sounds, identifying individual sounds in words, identifying and producing rhyming words, and blending sounds to make words.

Preferential seating: Where the student sits in the classroom that is close to where the teacher teaches, away from auditory and visual distractions, near a peer that can offer assistance, and/or increased distance between desks.

Rapid naming: The ability to quickly generate a list of like items (category).

Receptive vocabulary: Vocabulary that is understood.

Response to Intervention (RTI): A tiered scientific-based approach used to identify and provide intervention to students who may be struggling in certain academic areas or with behavior.

Section 504 of the Rehabilitation Act: Defines an individual with a disability. It states requirements for a free appropriate public education and appropriate modifications to support the students.

Semantics: The meaning or the interpretation of a word, sentence, or other language form.

Simile: A figure of speech that expresses a resemblance between things of different kinds usually formed with *like* or *as*.

Small group instruction: Teachers working with fewer students in the classroom for particular instruction in a specific area of learning.

Specially designed instruction: Defined in IDEA as adapting, as appropriate to the child's needs, the content, methodology, or delivery of instruction to address the unique needs of the student that result from the student's disability; to ensure access to the general education curriculum, so that the student can meet the educational standards within the jurisdiction of the public agency that apply to all students.

SQ3R: A reading comprehension strategy that employs the following steps: *Survey:* Scan the information; *Question:* Develop questions for each section; *Read:* Read the section; *Recite:* Answer the questions; *Review:* Go over one's notes.

Syntax: The rules that combine words or other elements of sentence structure to form grammatical sentences.

Title I: Title I of the Elementary and Secondary Education Act ensures that all students have a fair, equal opportunity to obtain a high-quality education regardless of status.

Validated screening system: Accurate in measuring and predicting improvements based on interventions provided.

Word finding: Difficulty retrieving words in single word context and discourse in the presence of good comprehension of the words that students are unable to find.

Working memory: Stores and manages the information required to carry out complex cognitive tasks such as learning, reasoning, and comprehension.

Index